DISCOVER YOUR

truebalance™

WITH

BIOIDENTICAL

HORMONES

Published by Advantage, Charleston, South Carolina.
Member of Advantage Media Group.

ADVANTAGE is a registered trademark and the Advantage colophon is a trademark of Advantage Media Group, Inc.

Printed in the United States of America.

ISBN: 978-1-59932-254-4
LCCN: 2011925217

This publication is designed to provide accurate and authoritative information in regard to the subject matter covered. It is sold with the understanding that the publisher is not engaged in rendering legal, accounting, or other professional services. If legal advice or other expert assistance is required, the services of a competent professional person should be sought.

Advantage Media Group is proud to be a part of the Tree Neutral® program. Tree Neutral offsets the number of trees consumed in the production and printing of this book by taking proactive steps such as planting trees in direct proportion to the number of trees used to print books. To learn more about Tree Neutral, please visit www.treeneutral.com. To learn more about Advantage's commitment to being a responsible steward of the environment, please visit www.advantagefamily.com/green

Advantage Media Group is a leading publisher of business, motivation, and self-help authors. Do you have a manuscript or book idea that you would like to have considered for publication? Please visit www.amgbook.com or call 1.866.775.1696

DISCOVERING YOUR

truebalance™

WITH

BIOIDENTICAL

HORMONES

DR. RON BROWN

Advantage®

A C K N O W L E D G E M E N T S

All books have a personal story to tell and this one is no exception. This book started with a question from a patient that started me on a path I would never have anticipated. Without that question and the circumstances that followed, there would be no book. I will be forever grateful to that patient, her name now forgotten, but her question never leaves me. Her question continues to push me on in directions I could not have predicted. I wish your face was as familiar to me as your question. Despite this, I am forever grateful for your ability to question conventional practice and your help letting me do the same. We truly live in marvelous times where skepticism and questioning can lead to incredible new ideas and truths. Thank you.

A book represents a significant investment of time and energy. It is not possible without many contributors and I would like to take a minute to thank those who helped make this book a reality. My first thanks, as is often the case, is to my spouse Susan. Susan is a natural entrepreneur, and over many years this outlook has rubbed off on me in small part. Susan also is able to make me better when it comes to refining practices in Bioidentical Hormone Replacement therapy. Her role as a nurse in the clinic always focuses our efforts on the patient. Her patience to let me spend the hundreds of hours necessary to research this book was invaluable. Without this time, the evidence to put this book on a firm foundation would not have been possible.

My next thank you is to my eldest son, David. David did much of the article collation, diagram preparation (as my computer skills are limited) and general illustrations. Thank you for the two summers of work that for this effort and the practitioner training manual required.

Anne Ryan believed in me and my vision from the start. She was able to see the "me" that I still have trouble seeing, and as such, was a large part of the genesis of this book.

Cheryl Antier was to be the ghost writer for this project. Despite her best efforts, it quickly became evident that this was a book that had to come from within me. Thank you Cheryl for your efforts, they were not in vain.

A big thanks needs to go to all the staff at True Balance. Korisa, my "superhero" assistant who runs the clinics and does most everything as it relates to BHRT. Norrie, Diane, Holly, Amy and all the other staff who make the clinic such a great place to work. Special thanks to the other practitioners at True Balance, who are always able to look at the problem from another perspective and give me insights beyond my own. Without all of these people and their contributions, this book would be much less than it is.

Thank you to my OBGYN partners, a never ending source of support. In these times it is easy to find people to criticize you, but seldom can you find such a remarkably supportive group. I have always known you were there to back me, even if what I was doing made no sense to you at all. Thank you again, Tom, Mike, Len and Carlissa-your presence in my corner was always felt.

Thank you to the two physicians who launched formal complaints to the Alberta College of Physicians and Surgeons. The angst and stress served to make me more committed and strong. Perhaps your intent was less than it should have been, but, the net result was a stronger and determined me. It is amazing what you can do with opposition and criticism when you feel in your heart that you are right.

Lastly, thank you to Brooke and the staff at Advantage Media Group. Right from the first interview, where Denis Boyles put me at ease and made the first supportive comments, I felt at home. Your team made the whole process painless to this "virgin author," and I am grateful.

If I have missed important contributors to this process, I apologize. Although I have failed to acknowledge you, I appreciate your assistance.

Thank You,

Ron Brown

Table of Contents

CHAPTER 1

INTRODUCTION

Why write another book on bioidentical hormones? I've asked myself this question sometimes on a day-to-day basis. (Especially at one in the morning, when I've struggled to get my thoughts down onto paper in a format that I hope you, my reader, will find entertaining and informative...or when I'm almost at the end of a 12-hour day, and I get an emergency call from a frantic husband whose wife is about to deliver their baby.)

The answer is, I'd like to give you greater insight into this area of medicine and, more importantly, into the possibilities and potential you have to live a longer, healthier, fuller life. So I'd like to start with a brief introduction, and tell you the story of how I came to be here, sitting at my old oak desk whenever I can carve out a few spare moments, to write this book for you. Because when it all boils down, that's why I'm doing it.

I believe that there is information about bioidentical hormone therapy, BHRT for short, that you need to know – to understand that there are real medical reasons for why you may not be feeling like your old self. Or, more accurately, like your younger self. Hormones are chemical messengers the body uses to adapt to outside factors. A hormone works on cells in tissues and organs of the body that have receptors for that hormone. We will go over this in more detail later, but a basic understanding will help set the stage for deeper understanding.

Hormone receptors are very specific three-dimensional structures, designed to bind a particular hormone. Until recently, hormones available for patient treatment were modified chemically to give them a different structure. Unfortunately, these modifications had far-ranging effects on the way these hormones work. This is a great story on unintentional consequences that I will go over in great detail. BHRT involves the use of human-identical hormones, or hormones with the EXACT molecular structure of the natural hormones they are meant to augment or replace. Use of bioidentical hormones allows a practitioner to replace or rebalance the patient's own hormones with ones that are identical to the original "real" hormones.

The imbalances and deficiencies of certain hormones that occur as we age, are the basis of many of the symptoms we experience as we get older, including low energy, anxiety, depression, insomnia, weight gain and memory loss, to name a few. BHRT allows us to correct the causes of these symptoms rather than using medications to mask or cover them up. This is the heart of why I am so passionate about BHRT, a passion I trust I will be able to convey and transfer to you.

And it's my hope that, as you read this book, you'll find the answers you've been looking for. I hope it validates your belief that what you've been going through ISN'T "all in your head" and that you don't just have to hope that if you ignore the symptoms long enough, they'll go away and someday you'll feel like your old self again. I hope it brings you to an understanding that you don't have to suffer in silence any more, or continue feeling powerless over what's going on in your body.

Because the fact is, none of that is true.

Throughout the book, you'll find descriptions of the most common symptoms for each of the hormonal imbalances, as well as what tests are recommended, and a little information about the latest, most cutting-edge treatment options.

In fact, that's one of the most important reasons I've spent the last several months writing this book – because I want you to understand that there **ARE** other options available to you besides those of conventional medicine. Instead of being told, "It's all in your head," or "Well, you have to expect this at your age, after all, you're not 20 years old now, you know," I want to reassure you that there are treatments other than the commonly prescribed pharmaceutical options, which only suppress one or more symptoms and force you to lead your life in a fog.

I want to give you enough information about your options so you're in the driver's seat and once again have the power and control over your health, your longevity, and, perhaps the most important of all, the power to regain your zest for living and to have the kind of life that you want and deserve.

ABOUT ME AND MY JOURNEY INTO BHRT

I have been a practicing obstetrician/gynecologist for the last 15 years. I am very fortunate to have the perfect job in Canada in this field. Right after medical school and a family medicine residency, I started practice as a country family doctor in Mundare, Alberta. For six years, I ran a small rural hospital and had a solo medical practice in this small town near Edmonton. They were special years because of the wonderful people I was fortunate to treat. However, after six years I knew I needed a change and decided to go into obstetrics and gynecology for the lifestyle! That may seem like a contradiction, but if you have ever been on call 24 hours a day, 365 days a year, you will know my perspective at the time! With the completion of my obstetrics residency, I started work in the Grey Nuns Hospital where I continue to practice as an Obstetrician/Gynecologist right up till today.

I've also had the privilege to work with a distinguished group of fellow Obstetrician/Gynecologists. They have been a great source of assistance, support and counsel. Obstetrics can be very stressful, and I've always appreciated and counted on having them in my corner. Many times an informal corridor consultation at the Grey Nuns Hospital – a premier provider of maternity and women's health services in Alberta – has helped improve the care of a patient. They have always given me the freedom within our practice to pursue my outside-the-box ideas and vision.

In fact, if things are so good in all aspects of the job, why venture into another area when demand for my services as an obstetrician far exceeds the time I can commit?

The answer will follow shortly.

But first, I'd like you to have an understanding of the path that brought me to this point. I have been married for 30 years to a wonderful partner, my wife, Susan. Over the years, I've come to believe that the best relationships serve to balance us. At least, that's the way it's worked for Susan and me.

Susan is a naturally gifted entrepreneur and has run an award-winning equestrian center for 35 years, and I respect and admire her abilities. Eight years ago, she talked me into starting a laser hair-removal company after a chance meeting with a salesperson in Toronto. At first, I objected to the idea. Didn't she realize that, as an obstetrician, I "knew" what women did and did not need? (It was my position back then that women did not have a problem with unwanted hair and therefore a laser hair-removal company was doomed to fail.)

Luckily for me, like many women, Susan didn't just listen to her husband and put away the idea. Instead, she did some market research. She discovered there was a demand for these services – and, almost in spite of me, a business was born. I'm happy to say that the company has continued to thrive – and it opened my eyes to the idea of private health-care services.

This is still a somewhat novel idea in a country of government-provided health care. If you're not familiar with the way medicine and health care works in Canada, it basically goes like this: A doctor sets up a practice and immediately has all the work he or she will ever need. In fact, a physician told me recently that she had to close her practice to new patients after only four months because she was too busy. Canada's supply of physicians has not kept up with the demands of our population growth – which means doctors are busier than they would like to be.

So you can see my point: With no limit on patient supply and guaranteed compensation from the government, why on earth would a busy physician need – or want – to look around for something else to do?

For me, this whole conundrum started with a patient whom I'm pretty sure all other doctors will recognize. I'm sorry to say that I can't remember her name, or her face, because my consultation with her started out like thousands of others. There was nothing remarkable or extraordinary about it. And yet, one simple question she asked ended up having a profound and immeasurable effect on my life.

It was a simple consultation for a hormone replacement in menopause. As was my normal procedure, I took a history, did an examination, and then, with a methodical approach, gave her the existing medical line on hormone replacement therapy – and by the way, the position of the medical establishment has not changed at all from that day. (I have confirmed this by attending a couple of recent talks on the subject where the status quo persists.) The status quo recommends the use of pharmaceutical hormones to relieve the symptoms of menopause. Unfortunately, these hormones are NOT for the most part, human identical, which leads to a number of serious problems in their use.

My patient politely listened to my carefully honed presentation on HRT and then asked what seemed to be an innocent question: What did I know about bioidentical hormone therapy? My answer was quick and factual. I didn't know anything about it.

Her response was equally rapid and to the point: Didn't it bother me, that as a specialist in women's health, I had no knowledge of this area of treatment? My response was again, short and to the point. "No." (I hadn't been a physician for 25 years without picking up a thing or two about how the medical consultation was supposed to go. She obviously didn't know that I was in charge of the interview – not her.)

That was the end of the consultation from her point of view, and she politely left. I never saw her again, but I trust she was able to find a practitioner who helped her with BHRT. But the effect of her question on me was much more unsettling and long-lasting. The implications of her question lingered. I would hear her voice in my head at odd moments. After a number of months, I decided that it did, in fact, bother me that there could be an area in my speciality that I was not completely knowledgeable about. I had heard through the medical grapevine that another obstetrician in my city was using bioidentical hormones.

However, since the mainstream conferences that I attend regularly have never discussed BHRT, I thought it had to be a fringe area. Even so, that little voice that kept slyly whispering in my ear, asking if it wouldn't be reasonable and responsible to attend a BHRT conference – just so that I could finally put this matter behind me?

And then another catalyst from an innocent-enough source happened around this same time: I read a book, *Fantastic Voyage*, by Dr. Terry Grossman and Ray Kurzweil, that completely changed the way I viewed this entire subject. (I don't know many people who can honestly say they've read a book that forever changed their lives, but it happened to me.)

The book was enthralling and eye-opening, especially as it pertains to how fast computer speed is growing and the capacity of computers to assimilate and process new information, and what that means to medicine in terms of accuracy and precision of tests and results. The basic premise of the book is that the rapid advances we see in computing speed and memory capacity have brought us to a point where we can start to grapple with the complexities of health.

They foresee transitions over the next few decades that will improve health and longevity beyond what can be imagined right now. One is already taking place, although we are largely unaware of it. It can be summed up as "The new 70 is the old 40." In other words, a 70-year-old today has the functional capacity and longevity of a 40-year-old in the middle of the last century. The exponential increase in computing power was seen with the Human Genome Project. This ambitious project to map the human genome was supposed to take 30 years, but took only eight, because of the rapid advance of testing abilities. Ray Kurzweil was alone in predicting this. In fact the next Archon Genomics X Prize will go to the team that can develop a test to map an individual's genome in 10 hours for less than $10,000. A reasonably priced test of one's genome will usher in a new degree of personalized medicine. Disease susceptibility on the basis of our genes will lead to specific hormone and nutritional recommendations to that individual aimed at avoidance of these diseases.

However, I have a conservative and analytical personality and I doubted many of the claims in the book. So I had my hospital library pull 100 or so of its references that pertained to the health field.

Every single one of the references supported the authors' conclusions, which was unsettling, because these articles were in the established scientific literature. So why were the recommendations for detailed testing and specific vitamin supplementation in these articles not making their way into the standard of practice guidelines?

Taking Grossman and Kurzweil's contentions to the next level led me to my colleagues. Internists and surgeons agreed that the medical literature supported their recommendations, but that they were not well enough established to change the current standard of care guidelines. It takes many years for new information to make it into clinical guidelines for patient treatment. Most medical doctors rely on these practice guidelines, especially when it involves changes to what they were taught.

The practice of medicine, you see, is very conservative. And while this has stood the profession in good stead over the centuries, I believe it is limiting in this day and age. As we move forward into ever-accelerating growth and innovation, conservatism no longer serves the profession or our patients well. Information about new medicines, new treatments, even breakthroughs is accumulating at an incredible speed, but the ability to move that new knowledge into clinical practice guidelines is not keeping up.

Ask a group of 20 business people, "How many of you use a BlackBerry/PDA for work?" and chances are all 20 will answer in the affirmative. The business world embraces technology and fast-paced changes to give it the competitive edge. But if you were to ask 20 physicians the same question, maybe four or five would say they do – and that's in even the most advanced of groups.

This will change with the next generation of physicians, but they are not the ones who write practice guidelines. Our professional structure and culture suppresses change and discourages innovation – and, sadly, I don't believe this will change anytime soon. We are in a time of incredible progress, but the institution of medicine is poorly equipped to embrace these changes. Individuals rely on physicians to be up to date with the most recent information. A large percentage of continuing medical education is dependant on financial support from the pharmaceutical industry. Disease treatment and prevention using nutrition and vitamins is the antithesis of the pharmaceutical model.

Is it not possible that this conflict of interest results in the preservation of the status quo? Most people I talk to would rather avoid disease and drug treatment if they had their choice. Prevention does little to help the bottom line of pharmaceutical companies, whose business model involves the use of medications on an ongoing basis, to treat the symptoms of certain disease processes. I will outline a number of strategies in this book to reduce the chance of disease manifestation in those who wish to take a proactive approach.

In any case, the next step in my own incredible journey led Susan and I to a longevity consultation with Dr. Grossman, coauthor of *Fantastic Voyage*, in Denver. Two days of sophisticated testing gave us a blueprint for our own personal health promotion and served as a springboard to my own professional development. He introduced me to directed vitamin supplementation as a means to delay or prevent development of disease.

Testing indicated areas of potential concern, such as excessive coronary artery calcification, and we developed strategies to reduce the chance of disease occurrence. Many of the diseases that conventional medicine regards as inevitable are, in fact, merely manifestations of vitamin and nutrient deficiencies. Coronary artery disease that eventually leads to heart attacks can be detected before significant blockage occurs. Niacin and Vitamin K are just two agents that can be used to halt and potentially reverse this process. Unfortunately, we have a medical industrial complex that has been built on the treatment of these diseases. What would happen to all the coronary angiogram suites, bypass surgery hospitals, and statin manufacturers if simple strategies were found to correct this disease process?

I am not a conspiracy theorist, but much more seems to be going on here than meets the eye. Bioidentical hormones seemed to fit in this world order of things, as a true preventative health strategy, and so I enrolled in my first BHRT conference. Many diseases that we encounter on a regular basis are a result of excessive inflammation. Treatment with bioidentical hormones can directly reduce inflammation and lead to a reduced chance of overt disease. Diseases of inflammation include diabetes, heart disease, Alzheimer's and cancer. Meanwhile, the question from that patient a year before continued to haunt me. I felt a new imperative. What did BHRT have to do with this whole area of developing medicine?

All of this fit into the context of running a full-time obstetrics and gynecology practice. This involves a 60- hour workweek and at least one night call thrown in for good measure. OB/GYNs are in short supply in Canada, and a night of being on-call is usually followed by a full day in the office – just to keep up with the demands of patient care.

My first BHRT conference, in Denver, was a significant milestone. Finally, I was introduced to the scientific side of BHRT. All treatment recommendations had supporting scientific information. The problem with this being a somewhat new area of medicine is that the available information is widely scattered and not well-organized. (This is a theme we will revisit in future sections of the book.)

I can't tell you how refreshing it was to be with a group of like-minded individuals. The majority of the practitioners at this conference were looking for answers, not just trying to preserve the status quo. Many medical practitioners have become fatalistic, believing that the present system is flawed, but not interested in pursuing other ideas. Here was a room full of people excited about the possibilities for a different approach to their patients' problems. The medical mix in the United States is more dynamic and innovative, due in large part to the influence of competition in its system. I do not see as much of this willingness to re-examine the tried-and-true approaches to health care in Canada. As of the writing of this book, I am not aware of any BHRT conferences in Canada. I hope to change that.

New concepts were introduced and discussed at length – in terms of present evidence in the scientific literature to support them. Much of this depends on the point of view one has when looking at the studies. In fact, it might interest you to know that both conventional hormone treatment and bioidentical hormone treatment camps can use the existing information to support their points of view.

I will try to give you my own perspective in this book as we journey together. I hope mine is a perspective of a practitioner with a foot firmly planted in both the conventional and nonconventional camps.

I remain a conventional obstetrician with an interest in some unconventional and emerging ideas. By the way, it's important to realize that all conventional treatment models were at one time unconventional and had to go through a process of displacing the existing treatments of the time.

I believe BHRT is at this stage right now.

After the conference, I went back to Canada and my conventional work. However, it was never the same old job after that. Suddenly, in my conventional practice, I began to see common threads with hormone deficiency and imbalance. These were treated with a combination of pharmaceutical agents, with or without surgery. Over time, I started to see that the BHRT approach could be used to make dramatic changes in patients as far as quality of life and even avoiding surgery.

I began to accumulate many hundreds of articles on BHRT and different aspects of longevity medicine. Many thanks go out to the librarians of my hospital, who never once complained of all the work I asked them to do. Gradually, with their help, I started to put together a very complete set of reference works to provide supporting evidence to BHRT.

The next stop on this voyage was a conference hosted by the American Academy of Anti-Aging Medicine (A4M). This is a young but vibrant association devoted to the study and promotion of longevity medicine. I was introduced to innumerable concepts and a whole new area to pursue. The A4M has an organized and accredited fellowship in Functional and Regenerative Medicine. Although it seemed like the last thing I needed to add to my schedule, there was really no question about whether to proceed.

After extensive preparation, I passed the exams and completed the A4M fellowship. I remain deeply indebted to the Academy and Dr. Pam Smith for the content of the program. Huge amounts of work went into its organization, with Dr. Smith doing the lion's share. All evidence produced required at least two articles of confirmation in the conventional medical literature in order for it to be included in the course material.

But, as you can imagine, there is not a lot of free time left over, after all of these activities and a full-time OB/GYN practice. Which is why I must mention the sacrifices my family – my wife, Susan; and children Ashley, David, Ryan and Daena – has made to allow me to pursue this interest. I am deeply grateful to all of them for their support and encouragement. Without it, this book would never have seen the light of day. Susan, the entrepreneur, has slowly molded my mindset and thoughts to allow me to see the possibilities, not the obstacles. Without her input and energy, BHRT would have remained an interesting area with little relevance to the real world for me.

WHAT'S HAPPENING NOW

At the end of the fellowship, an interesting conversion started to take place in my life and my practice. First was the development of a private BHRT practice with full availability of "patient pay" testing. (Some of the testing for BHRT does not exist in the government-sponsored system in Canada.) I made lab contacts, ordered tests, and developed office systems.

Many thanks to Korisa Homan, my indispensible Girl Friday for bioidentical hormones, and all her hard work in this regard. It can be challenging to implement the ideas of a busy boss who is difficult to track down and always trying to be in two places at once. In fact, this process was successful only because a private office practice already existed that allowed its development. And word-of-mouth brought patients to our door, which allowed me to continue and build a BHRT practice.

The regular OB/GYN practice continued to provide examples appropriate to BHRT and streamlining of the process on the clinical side. As my experience grew, some of my talents came to the forefront. I have always been a systems person and that approach led to ever-improving results and more word-of-mouth referrals. What started as one day a week has led to two days a week of exclusive BHRT practice.

All of this is somewhat unusual in Canada, the land of free health care, as all these patients are private-pay. It is complicated and time-intensive to do BHRT well – and those elements do not lend themselves to the government system. What at first seemed to be an obstacle turned out to be an advantage. An existing private laser hair removal business turned out to be the ideal place to start a private bioidentical hormone practice.

Even in a public system, patients will pay for an approach that is consistent with their own goals. At its heart, BHRT remains a preventive medical approach that is quite at odds with the present-day disease treatment model. I will have much more to say about this in later chapters as well.

A reasonable system has led to the inclusion of other practitioners. I am deeply indebted to the courageous Dr. Marichal Binns, Dr. Cynthia Olson and Dr. Heather Reese. It takes a lot of personal bravery to step out of the conventional mold and set yourself apart professionally. In that process, these individuals showed how this BHRT system can serve more than one practitioner. Those in the established system seem inclined to take shots at physicians willing to look at and explore new areas.

I believe the words of John Maxwell, a writer looking at the effects of change in our lives, illustrates our present situation. "The difficulty lies not so much in developing new ideas as in escaping from the old ideas. Until we get used to living with something that is not comfortable, we cannot get any better." These words ring true for the present situation with BHRT.

Longevity medicine and BHRT are really just a form of a personalized, preventive health program fully supported by scientific research.

Have all the questions been answered? No, of course not. But the process is under way and requires our support if it is to be fully realized. And I am excited and honoured to be a part of it – in fact, I'm more excited about this area of medicine than any other I have been involved with in more than 25 years of practice – and that is no small feat.

In the pages that follow, I am going to try to share my sense of excitement and hope developed over three years of working with BHRT. As one patient said to me, quite succinctly, "This area is all about hope. With the use of this therapy, you have given me my life back. Thank you."

For more inforamtion on Medical Grade Aesthetics and Bioidentical Hormone Replacement Therapy (BHRT), please visit my website at:

mytruebalance.ca

CHAPTER 2

WHAT ARE HORMONES AND BIOIDENTICAL HORMONES?

Hormones are the chemical messengers that communicate between one part of the body and another. They are produced by an organ and then secreted into the bloodstream where they circulate. Hormones diffuse out of the blood vessels into the various tissues of the body. Only tissues with receptors to a particular hormone will respond to that hormone. Really, when you think about it, the body has developed an amazing system over the evolutionary process. Everything the body does is designed to maintain homeostasis, or a stable environment, which allows it to function properly. Hormones are one of the main tools the body uses to maintain homeostasis.

The body's method of interfacing with the outside environment is generally controlled through the central nervous system. That's why many of the glands that secrete hormones are controlled from centers in the brain. The senses of sight, sound, pain, touch and taste convey aspects of the external environment to the brain. Different areas of the brain are responsible for a particular sense and the processing of information for that sense.

These brain centers monitor both internal and external body environments and, when necessary, send messages to specific glands that produce specific hormones. The type and amount of hormone that needs to be produced depends on the environment being sensed by the brain centers – but the directions for its production is very precise.

Once secreted into the bloodstream, these hormones circulate both in both free form and tied to hormone-binding-proteins, or globulins, as well as red blood cell membranes. The sex hormones that are not free, represent up to 97% of the hormone in blood and circulate bound to sex-hormone binding globulin (SHBG) and albumin. These bound hormones are not available to tissues and form a reservior of the hormone in the bloodstream. This reservior serves to even out hormone surges and dips, all in aid of homeostasis. The free hormone is able to diffuse out of the blood vessels, into the cells of the tissues. If the hormone molecule reaches a cell with its particular receptor, hormone-receptor binding occurs. For the sex hormones, receptor binding occurs in the nucleus of the cell. Receptor binding initiates a cellular response, usually resulting in the production of a protein that directs the function of the cell. Only cells with receptors for a particular hormone will respond to that hormone. This is the way the body controls what tissues respond to a particular hormone.

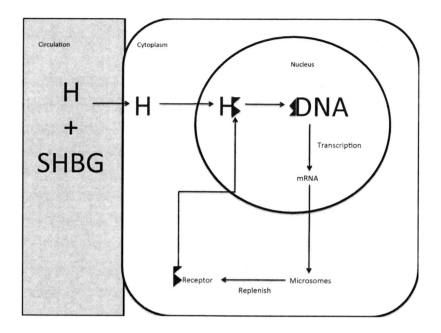

Fig. 2-1: Hormone Receptor Action

Bioidentical hormone therapy (BHRT) is mostly focused on the replacement of the primary sex hormones: estrogen, progesterone and testosterone.

We will be discussing a number of the other important body hormones, such as cortisol and thyroid hormone in this book. Thyroid and adrenal function are critical for the proper function of the sex hormones. These hormones work in a slightly different fashion than the sex hormones. Their control and function is complicated and beyond the scope of this book. But one of the most important things for you, the reader, to know, is that if there is a disturbance in thyroid or adrenal function, all hormone systems will be negatively affected.

However, most of our discussion will center on the sex hormones, as they are principal ingredients of well-being.

As a gynecologist, I feel well qualified to speak about these hormones. Their changes as we age cause much of the reduced quality of life we experience.

All of the hormones we're going to talk about are steroid hormones. These include estrogen, progesterone, testosterone and cortisol. The body manufactures steroid hormones from cholesterol, which is the basic chemical backbone. The chart below shows how the body does so. Note that estriol production from estrone is a one-way street; estriol can't be converted back to estrone. This is an important fact that contributes to the safety of estriol in the body.

Men and women share all of these hormones; the only difference is in the absolute and relative amounts to one another.

Let's look at each class in a little more detail, because in order to understand BHRT, you have to have a basic understanding of each of the types of hormones, what their purpose and function are, and what happens to them as we age or are exposed to stress and environmental stimuli.

ESTROGENS

This book has been written primarily for women, and estrogen is the primary hormone we think of when considering the female condition. The adrenal glands and ovaries produce estrogen, with each being responsible for roughly 50% of the production in premenopausal women.

Estrogen receptors are widely distributed throughout the body in areas such as the brain, breast, bone, blood vessels and reproductive organs. Estrogens are critical for sexual maturation, puberty and the reproductive cycle. Adult women produce three primary estrogens: estradiol, extrone and estriol.

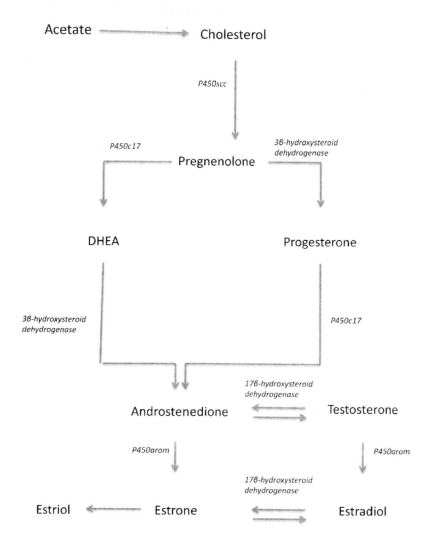

Fig. 2-2: Hormone Pathways

ESTRADIOL

Estradiol is the strongest of the estrogens and the main one produced by the ovaries. It is the primary estrogen of the menstrual cycle and is responsible for building up the thickness of the uterine lining in preparation for egg implantation. Approximately 50% of estradiol production comes from the ovaries. The rest starts with adrenal production of a hormone called androstenedione, which is then converted in the tissues to estradiol and estrone (a weaker estrogen).

Estradiol production varies throughout the menstrual cycle, as the diagram illustrates. Remember, hormones have significant effects on mood and thought. The brain has the highest level of estrogen receptors of all the organs in the body. Is it any wonder that changes in estrogen cause mood disturbances?

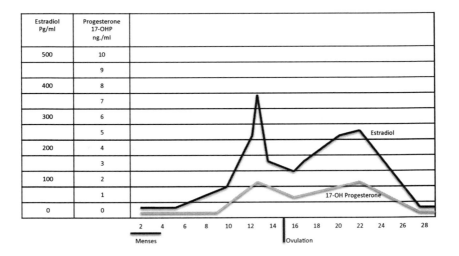

Fig. 2-3: Hormone levels during the menstrual cycle

The hormonal foundations of the emotions in women are forever changing. As you can see, the balance of estrogen and progesterone shifts back and forth through the monthly menstrual cycle. Disturbances in this ratio can lead to anxiety, emotional outbursts and insomnia. After many years of observation I can clearly and emphatically state that a woman's emotional symptoms are NEVER in her head! In a woman's 30s and 40s, estradiol production is relatively steady, while progesterone steadily falls over this time period. This imbalance is so important that I will devote an entire chapter to it. Estrogen dominance is truly one of the epidemics of our time.

Estradiol production becomes erratic in the late 40s with surges and falls, until it finally falls dramatically with the onset of menopause. And, of course, very low levels of estrogen produce a whole new set of symptoms for women to deal with in menopause, which we'll explore further in future chapters.

ESTRONE

Estrone is the next strongest estrogen and is produced by conversion of estradiol in the tissues. Estrone is the main post-menopausal estrogen and can be converted to either estradiol or estriol, if required. Estrone can also be conjugated to estrone sulphate in the liver. Conjugation allows estrone to be stored in a safe fashion and also lets the body excrete it as needed to maintain proper balance. More than half of the body's estrogen is stored as estrone sulphate. In this form, it cannot bind to the estrogen receptor but it can be converted into estradiol

ESTRIOL

Estriol is the weakest of the three natural estrogens. This is important to remember, because it is used extensively in BHRT treatments. Normally, estriol is produced in high levels only during pregnancy and it seems to have important functions in both pregnancy support and breast cancer protection. Estriol acts to block the potent effects of estradiol on breast-tissue growth and possible cancer promotion.

Studies have shown that the more estriol a woman produces during pregnancy (and the younger she is with her first pregnancy and the more pregnancies she has), the lower her lifetime risk for breast cancer. BHRT uses this weak estrogen as part of an overall strategy to reduce breast cancer risk. A product called Biest is the most commonly prescribed BHRT transdermal estrogen, and it contains both estradiol and estriol.

PROGESTERONE

Progesterone is the natural antagonist, or balancer, to estrogen. We can think of estrogen and progesterone as the yin and yang of the female hormone system. Their relative balance determines either a state of physical and emotional well-being or unpleasant symptoms. Progesterone is essential for maintenance of pregnancy and is also the principal hormone of the luteal phase, or second half, of the menstrual cycle.

The first half of the menstrual cycle is called the follicular stage. It is characterized by high levels of estrogen as the body prepares the endometrial lining of the uterus for implantation of the fertilized egg. The luteal phase, or second half, is characterized by high levels of progesterone, which support the implantation of the egg, should conception take place. If there is no conception, the abrupt drop in progesterone levels at the end of this phase results in the menstrual period.

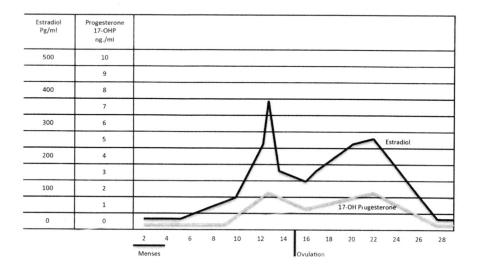

Fig. 2-4: Hormone levels during the menstrual cycle

Even within the menstrual cycle, progesterone is the natural balance to estrogen. Chronically poor progesterone levels put women at risk of disorders such as fibroids, endometriosis and uterine cancer, illustrating how well-being and health depend on achieving balance in these two sex hormones.

Progesterone is produced naturally by the ovaries after ovulation, as well as by the brain and adrenal glands in small measure. Progesterone receptors are found throughout the body, in the brain, breasts, blood vessels, bones and reproductive organs. There must be a reason nature put progesterone receptors in these areas. Which brings me to hysterectomy.

If you've had a hysterectomy, you know that the removal of your uterus does not change all the tissues' basic need for progesterone to function properly or the brain's requirement for it. With respect to progesterone, a woman is much more than a uterus, and this has been sadly overlooked in the typical medical approach. I hope to help convince you this oversight is incorrect and harmful.

TESTOSTERONE

Testosterone is not just a male hormone, though that's the common perception – which is probably why it has been much overlooked in women's health. I predict we will see this change over the next five to 10 years.

In women, testosterone is critical to the optimal functioning of many of systems. Sex drive, heart health, the preservation of bone and muscle mass – as well as a sense of well-being – are all improved with the correction of deficient testosterone levels.

Women's bodies produce only 10% of the testosterone produced by males, but that 10% is critical to good health. Testosterone production falls by 50% from age 20 to 40 and continues to fall until menopause. It drops even further during pregnancy. Each successful term pregnancy results in a 10% to 15% further fall in testosterone production. This is truly nature's family planning method – the more pregnancies a woman has, the less testosterone she produces, resulting in a lower sex drive. Less sex means less children, who says Nature doesn't know what she is doing?

In addition, testosterone in overweight women can be converted to estrogen in fat tissue by a process termed aromatization. And this can result in a further drop in testosterone levels.

In a future chapter we will look at the syndrome of testosterone deficiency and how pervasive it has become today, as well as what you can do if you suspect you have this condition.

After menopause, testosterone production stabilizes and levels no longer fall. Since estrogen production has fallen dramatically in this period, there is relative testosterone excess as it relates to estrogen, even though overall testosterone levels are low. Post-menopausal women may see the results of this in the form of a discernible moustache.

But remember, it's all about the balance among these hormones – and that's what this book will help you figure out for your own health and well being.

CORTISOL

Cortisol is the basic hormone of survival and is released by the adrenal glands. It is not a sex hormone, but it's so important that it deserves mention.

Cortisol is responsible for the fight-or-flight response which, as we know, served our ancestors well in avoiding the odd sabre-toothed tiger or other deadly threat they came across – it was thanks to cortisol's actions that they could run faster, think quicker, and avoid becoming the entrée du jour on the lunch menu. However, once they were no longer at risk for being eaten, the stress went away and life went back to normal.

Although we generally don't have to worry about being something's lunch these days, we have different, but equally serious, problems to deal with – which means stress appears in many different forms in our daily lives and has become chronic. We were never designed to handle ongoing stress, and the chronic stress of these modern times has led to some serious health issues for a large part of the population. Because cortisol is the survival hormone, it trumps all the other hormones – who cares about reproduction if you are going to be lunch, right?

Cortisol is very responsive to emotional stress and has a number of important functions. It increases the release of sugar in to the bloodstream, defends against infection and inflammation, and regulates the effects of the other hormones. Stressful factors in our lives – a bad boss, difficult job, marital difficulties, challenges with our children and finances – can increase our cortisol levels, which has a negative effect on our health and well being, and actually can put us on the track of accelerated aging.

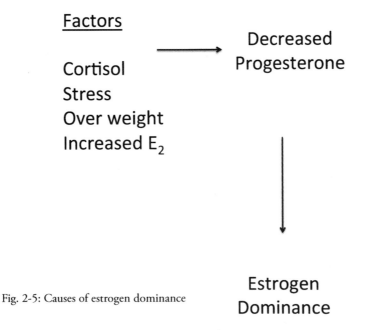

Factors

Cortisol
Stress
Over weight
Increased E_2

Decreased
Progesterone

Estrogen
Dominance

Fig. 2-5: Causes of estrogen dominance

Progesterone is the natural chill pill and modulates the effects of excess cortisol. As progesterone levels fall from age 30 to 50, our ability to handle stress declines. BHRT always addresses the functional lack of progesterone and leads to a reduction in factors contributing to premature aging.

HORMONES AND WEIGHT GAIN

Cortisol increases blood sugar levels and make it more difficult for insulin to facilitate entry of glucose into the cells of the body. The body responds with higher insulin levels and an increased tendency to gain weight.

High levels of cortisol also inhibit the production of active thyroid hormone. Thyroid hormone is responsible for out metabolic rate and a reduction in its activity leads to weight gain and lower energy levels. The end result is that chronic stress causes us to gain weight. As we age, stress tends to increase and so does that number on the scale. *Complete coincidence? I think not!*

Because cortisol is so powerful, the body has several natural cortisol antagonists whose job are to keep it in balance. We have already seen that progesterone declines from age 25 to 50, even in the face of rising cortisol levels. The other cortisol antagonist is called DHEA (dehydro-epiandrostendione). However, DHEA production peaks at age 25 and declines to only 10% of that level by age 80.

As DHEA declines, its balance with cortisol decreases and the negative effects of excess cortisol begin accumulating. The balance between androgenic hormones (testosterone and DHEA) and cortisol also helps preserve muscle mass. Androgens build muscle while cortisol tears it down. As we age, our androgen levels fall, cortisol levels rise and the net result is our muscles begin to break down. And as muscle mass erodes, our metabolic rate decreases, making it possible to gain weight without increasing calorie intake.

Cortisol stimulates aromatase activity and increases estrogen levels. Remember, aromatase converts testosterone and other androgens to estrogen, and while some estrogen is good, you can get too much of a good thing. Cortisol also competes with progesterone at its receptor level and produces a functional deficiency of progesterone. *(Which is why when being tested for progesterone deficiency, your overall progesterone secretion could be in the normal range, but high cortisol levels make it look like there is too little progesterone when we look at a symptom chart.)* The net effect of these two actions is to create an estrogen dominance pattern that is associated with a tendency to gain weight.

And increased weight causes increased aromatase activity and more conversion of androgens and testosterone to estrogens, starting a vicious circle – stress, estrogen dominance, weight gain, more stress, etc.

If this all seems kind of complicated, just remember that the end result of chronic stress is more weight gain and more fat tissue – and the start of a vicious cycle that means the older you get, the harder it can be to lose weight – and the easier it is to gain weight – even if you haven't changed your eating habits. It also means it has little to do with self-control and willpower, and is the real reason why diets and exercise don't give you the results you want.

By now you're no doubt beginning to have a much clearer picture of how your overall health, well-being – and even your emotions – are controlled by the balance of a number of powerful hormones.

HOW BHRT CAN HELP

With BHRT, we can correct the cortisol/androgen ratio to preserve and build muscle mass. This, in turn, leads to healthier aging and the reduced chance of disease. It can also help to increase metabolism, increase your body's ability to process natural insulin, and stabilize weight gain.

Here's something else you need to understand in order to take control of your health and be a part in the decision-making process of your medical treatment: In the medical establishment, different fields of medicine have staked out their territory on the different hormones and the treatment plans. (Think of it as two kids playing King of the Hill. Each wants to be the king, and neither one is willing to back down or share the hill.)

For example, gynecology "owns" estrogen, progesterone and testosterone. Endocrinology "controls" cortisol, growth hormone, DHEA and thyroid hormones. Each field is a kind of law unto itself and, as a general rule, is not used to playing nice with the others. I have only recently seen an endocrinologist at a BHRT conference and I have never attended an endocrinology conference.

BHRT could be the referee that brings everyone together. It represents an attempt to unify the two groups to create a better understanding of how these hormones all act in concert. This understanding can help each area of medicine give patients the best possible health and quality of life as they get older.

The emphasis and focus of this book is about the balance of hormones. "Absolute levels" of hormones are really just an illusion that is holding us back. The number of a hormone level is much less important than the ratio of it to its hormone partners.

And that's where BHRT shines. Only by understanding how hormones work, how they interact with one another, and how they balance one another, can we improve health in a fundamental way. It's an area that has always been of great interest to me, an interest which has only gotten stronger as my journey into BHRT has continued.

Pathophysiology is the study of the basic mechanisms of disease development. It allows us to see why something goes wrong in the body and produces a disease – diabetes, for example.

And here's why this is so fascinating to me: Once we understand the basic hormonal imbalances that created the disease, we can start reversing those effects and move toward eliminating those diseases. That's much different from the present approach of using medication on a permanent basis to treat the symptoms, but cover up the disease. Most people I talk to would rather rid themselves of a disease, rather than simply using medication as a Band-aid to reduce the symptoms.

You've probably heard of miners using canaries to warn of imminent danger. Methane was a silent, odorless and deadly killer in the early coalmines. Since it was undetectable, miners devised a simple solution. They carried these fragile birds in cages down into the mines. If the canary keeled over, it was time to get everyone out to safety.

Patient symptoms are the canary in the coal mine of hormone imbalances. Once we start paying attention to them – and their level of severity – I believe we can prevent the problems from occurring in the first place. The chart below is the symptom list I use in my BHRT practice. Patients score their symptoms at EACH visit to ensure we are making progress on their quality of life. BHRT really is all about the patient and their concerns!

Your Hormone Balance Inventory

		0	5	10	15	20
		None	Slightly	Moderate	Severe	Extreme
Progesterone						
If your scoring is between 20 and 30 in this sections you may be deficient in progesterone	Difficulty Concentrating					
	Moodiness/ Emotional Swings					
	Depressed or Unhappy					
	Anxious					
	Headaches					
	Can't Sleep (Insomnia)					
	Painful or Swollen Breasts					
	Weight Gain/ Bloating					
	PMS					
Estrogen						
If your Scoring is between 20 and 30 in this section you may need Estrogen supplementation	Night Sweats					
	Difficulty Remembering Things					
	Hot Flashes					
	Vaginal Dryness					
	Dry Hair/ Skin					
	Incontinence					
	Frequent Urinary Tract Infection					
	Inability to Reach Orgasm					
	Painful Intercourse					
Testosterone						
If any item is checked in this area you may need Testosterone	Loss of Libido					
	Lack of Desire to be in Intimate					
	Loss of Motivation					
	Flat Mood					
	Diminished Well Being					
	Blunted Motivation					

Table 2-1 Hormone inventory

HOW IT WORKS

When the brain sends a message to a gland, a hormone is produced and secreted into the bloodstream, where it circulates throughout the body, and is distributed to the all tissues. The tissues that need that hormone for proper function have receptors for that specific hormone. Hormone-receptor binding starts the production of proteins within the cell and a change in cell function or status. Translate this to the entire organ and we see a difference in the function of that organ.

Hormones are secreted in pulses that produce significant ranges of normal values. This fact has always held back the study of hormones, because they produce a high signal-to-noise ratio. The range of normal for a hormone secreted in a pulse fashion is so wide that even people with dramatic hormone imbalances can have hormone levels within the normal range. It is only when hormones are interpreted in terms of their balance, along with patient symptoms, that a clear picture starts to emerge.

Our bodies regulate the hormonal messages they send and receive based on a number of factors (such as stress, certain drugs, environmental exposures or aging). It's a kind of Morse code, designed to regulate the amount of hormones being secreted – or made available to the tissues. As well, by binding the hormones to carrier proteins in the blood the net effect is to smooth out the hormone message being sent to the body. Once the hormones are bound, they can't diffuse out of the bloodstream into target tissues. Instead, they act as a kind of reservoir to even out the pulses of hormone production and give the body a more regulated level of a particular hormone.

But the levels of the different binding proteins are not fixed — they can be altered by prescription drugs and hormone imbalances. This has very important implications when we look at the effects of different forms of hormone replacement and their resulting actions on the hormone carrier protein levels.

Let's look at the sex hormones for example: The main carrier protein in the blood for testosterone, estrogen and progesterone is a protein called sex-hormone binding globulin (SHBG). Sex-hormone binding globulin is produced by the liver and strongly binds the sex hormones as they circulate in the blood. (And remember, when a hormone is bound to SHGB, it's not available to the tissues.)

While it binds all the sex hormones, SHBG has a preference for testosterone. Estrogen, when taken as a pill, dramatically increases the production of SHBG by the liver. That means taking estrogen in pill form leaves a smaller amount of free testosterone that can be used to regulate the body and get rid of specific symptoms related to menopause. There is also less free testosterone to balance out estrogen and prevent anxiety and moodiness.

There is another, weaker binding protein or globulin for sex hormones called albumin. It has a high affinity but low binding power and therefore the hormones are only loosely associated with it, making them more available to the tissues. Only about 1% to 2% of all hormones are considered free or unbound and therefore available to the tissues.

One more method of hormone transport is not completely understood. Red blood cells (RBCs) are able to transport large amounts of hormone through the blood. In fact, some researchers believe they are like hormone super-tankers. This may be very important for hormones that are rubbed on the skin, such as with transdermal treatment (application of cream to the skin) used with BHRT. Hormones are weakly bound to RBCs and therefore very available to the tissues. This may explain why transdermal estrogen and testosterone are so effective in the relief of hormone-deficiency symptoms.

HORMONE MEASUREMENT

Your physician needs to know the type of measurement used to check a hormone level in the blood. There are several different methods, such as:

- *Total hormone:* All bound and freely circulating hormone levels in the blood. Not that accurate, because it can be influenced by the amounts of SHBG and albumin.

- *Bioavailable hormone:* Measures free and albumin-bound hormone levels. More accurate for the clinical picture, but requires measurement of SHBG and albumin levels. It is less accurate than free hormone levels.

- *Free hormone:* Hormones circulate in the blood in both free and bound form. It is only the free fraction that is available to leave the circulation and diffuse into the interstitial fluid, the fluid between the cells.

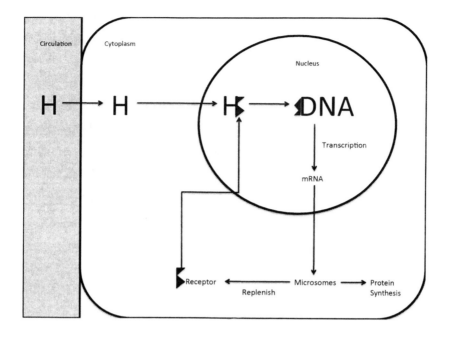

Fig. 2-6: Hormone receptor action

This diagram above shows a free hormone leaving the bloodstream, diffusing into the cell, and binding to its receptor. Once the key fits into the receptor lock, it initiates a response within the nucleus of the cell where the hormone receptor resides – just the way a key turns in a lock to open the door. After its effect, the hormone is removed from the nucleus and either removed from the cell, broken down or recycled (replenished).

Different types of tissue, such as heart, bone and uterus, respond to the same hormone in the same fashion. What action the hormone produces is determined by the presence and concentration of a particular hormone receptor within that tissue. Hormone and receptor coupling, followed by DNA binding, initiates the same protein production in all tissues with the hormone receptor. No receptor, no action. It's that simple. Receptor distribution and density is responsible for the different actions of different tissues with the same concentration of hormones. Perhaps nature had a purpose in placing the receptors that is beyond the simple ways we look at things today.

This next area is a little technical, but bear with me, because it's important. All sex hormones consist of an 18 to 20 carbon structure with a specific structure called a perhydrocyclopentanophenanthrene molecule, made up of three 6-carbon rings and one 5-carbon ring. Its exact composition gives this particular steroid molecule its unique three-dimensional shape. And it's this three-dimensional shape that gives each steroid its receptor specificity – just like a specific key is only made for a specific lock.

All steroid hormones are made from cholesterol as the initial building block. Different enzymes work on cholesterol to form the different steroid molecules (Fig. 2-7, below). As we can see from the figure, pregnenolone is the "mother" hormone.

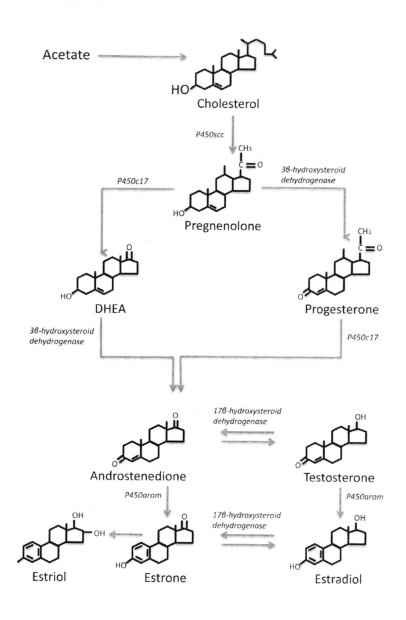

Fig. 2-7: Hormone composition

Pregnenolone is converted to progesterone and DHEA (dehydroepiandrosterone) in hormone-producing tissues in the body. Next comes androstenedione, which is used to make testosterone and estrone. Estradiol is the final product in this synthesis pathway, as illustrated in the diagram.

As you can see, each one of these hormones has a very specific three-dimensional shape, which gives its hormone receptor specificity. This is a key concept and cannot be over-emphasized. All hormones are not created equal. This is particularly true of hormones modified by the pharmaceutical industry to comply with patent law. A progestin is a chemical modification of progesterone and does not necessarily have all of the attributes of progesterone. We will discuss this at length in Chapter 8.

NATURAL HORMONES VS. HUMAN-IDENTICAL HORMONES

Bioidentical hormones are synthetics that have the identical molecular structure to the ones the body produces. For the most part, they are made from diogensin, a compound that is very similar to cholesterol – which we know is where the body starts when it wants to make a steroid hormone. Diogensin is found in high concentrations in the Mexican yam. Through a series of chemical reactions, it can be converted into estrogen, progesterone and testosterone.

Bioidentical hormones ARE NOT NATURAL! There is NOTHING natural about the synthetic processes used to convert diogensin to the sex hormones. To say otherwise is false and part of the problem that conventional medicine has with claims made regarding bioidentical hormones. Untrue claims regarding the "natural" status of bioidentical hormones have helped to form a barrier to their acceptance by conventional medicine. This issue has become a lightning rod to focus the discontent regarding the new approach to disease and patient symptoms. Bioidentical hormones represent part of a new approach to health care and many elements of conventional health care find this very threatening. So far it has been easier to focus on this obvious inaccuracy than to deeply examine the problems with the existing approach to health care. We urgently need to change from a disease-treatment system to that of a health-optimization approach. The longer the two camps continue to argue about who is right, the longer this refocusing will take.

The fact is that these BHRT products are "human identical," a term coined by Dr. Jonathon Wright, meaning that they are identical to their natural human counterparts on a molecular level and have all of the properties of the natural hormones.

Up to now, the advancement and recognition of BHRT has been held back by false claims of "natural" and "safe." BHRT steroids are no more harmful and no safer than the natural hormones. Imbalances in our natural hormones can cause disease, just as those same imbalances in bioidentical hormones can. We will explore in detail why bioidentical hormones have some significant advantages over synthetic hormones in terms of safety. The absolute levels and balance between hormones creates "safety" or "potential danger," and that's a fact that must never be forgotten.

Now that we know what hormones and bioidentical hormones are, we are ready to explore why there is a problem in the first place. A basic knowledge of hormones is a prerequisite for understanding why imbalances and resulting symptoms occur.

Important Points

1. The brain senses changes in the internal and external environment through the senses and their associated brain centers.

2. The brain regulates hormone production to allow the body to adapt to changes in the internal and external environment.

3. Sex hormones are one group of hormones whose production is under control of the brain.

4. Proper balance of certain sex hormone pairs is critical to proper body function: estrogen/progesterone and estrogen/testosterone are 2 of the very important pairs for BHRT.

5. Hormone levels change with age and other factors, such as weight gain and pregnancy.

6. Chronic stress increases cortisol levels. We live in very stressful times as a society.

7. Increased cortisol interferes with the normal function of sex hormones.

8. An increased cortisol/sex hormone ratio leads to breakdown in muscle mass and body metabolism.

9. Hormones are three-dimensional molecules whose exact structure is responsible for their specific action in the target cell.

10. Bioidentical hormones are NOT natural, they are created synthetically.

11. Bioidentical hormones are "human identical" and work exactly like the body's own hormones if prescribed in proper balance.

12. Hormone balance is more important than hormone levels.

CHAPTER 3

WHY DO WE HAVE A PROBLEM WITH HORMONES?

In a perfect world, we would all have a perfect metabolism, a stress-free lifestyle, and harmless environmental factors. Our bodies would continue to function as well as they did in our 20s as we got older.

But, sadly, that's not the way things are. Once we reach our mid-20s, it's all downhill – at least from a hormonal standpoint. Conventional medicine would have us believe it's just a coincidence that we experience the best health of our lives during our 20s.

You'll probably agree that back then, you had boundless energy and a metabolism that let you get away with many indiscretions when it came to your diet or cutting back on sleep – with no apparent adverse effects. But the older you got, the harder it became to drop a few pounds after over-indulging during the holidays, or while you were on vacation, or after those little late-afternoon sugary snacks that you needed for a quick pick-me-up. And gradually, it took more than dieting over the weekend or doing a little extra exercise to get rid of those few extra pounds.

You probably have noticed the same thing about sleep. If you partied all night when you were younger, you could make it up by sleeping in late on Sunday morning, or going to bed early for a few nights during the week. And you'd wake up feeling refreshed and raring to go.

And again, the older you got, the harder it was to catch up on sleep – in fact, you might have started having a hard time sleeping through the night – and when you got up in the mornings, more often than not, you felt more tired than you did when you went to bed.

It was easier when you were younger because of the amounts and balance of hormones. It's harder now because of the overall lower levels of hormones and some imbalances between hormones.

In this chapter, we're going to go over how our hormone production declines over time. And we're going to review environmental and lifestyle issues as they pertain to hormone production

ESTROGEN

As we discussed in Chapter 1, a woman's estrogen production (compared with the other sex hormones) is well-maintained until peri-menopause. Most women will enter peri-menopause in their mid-40s, although this varies greatly from one woman to another.

During this peri-menopause period, women often develop wild fluctuations in estrogen secretion. Sometimes you may experience estrogen surges, followed by times when estrogen production falls remarkably. This can result in a variety of symptoms and emotions, or feeling as if something's "off," and yet you're not really able to explain or pinpoint exactly what's wrong. (This is normal, and you're not alone.)

In general, however, your overall estrogen secretion is reasonably maintained until the onset of menopause. Then, during menopause, your estrogen production falls dramatically and does not recover. This is often accompanied by an onset of symptoms including hot flashes and flushes, vaginal dryness, and decreased concentration and memory, to name just a few.

Diagnosis of menopause actually happens after the fact: Doctors diagnose it after a woman has had no menstrual bleeding for 12 months. These changes in estrogen production are well-illustrated in the chart below showing hormone production over a woman's lifetime.

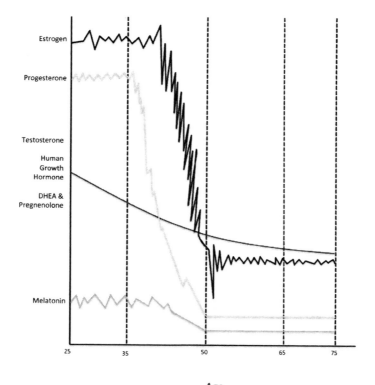

Fig. 3-1: Hormone-production decline over age

During a woman's child-bearing years, the pituitary gland in the brain secretes FSH (follicle stimulating hormone) to stimulate development of the egg and estrogen secretion. As estrogen secretion falls, the FSH will gradually rise – an indication that the brain centers are trying to push the ovaries to produce more estrogen.

Complicated feedback loops from the ovary to the brain are in place to ensure proper levels of estrogen secretion are maintained. As estrogen production falls through the menopausal transition as a result of ovarian failure, FSH levels rise as menopause establishes itself. In fact, an FSH level above 30 mmol/l is used to make the presumptive diagnosis of menopause. FSH will rise before periods actually stop, as the brain tries to get the ovaries to work harder when it senses lower estrogen levels.

The ovarian follicles produce estrogen, primarily estradiol, as they develop each month. During each cycle, hundreds or more follicles will start to develop and a complicated kind of hormone competition takes place. Estrogen is the only hormone with the ability to up-regulate, or increase, the number of its own receptors. It is also the only hormone that can recycle itself – through a process called replenishment.

These special abilities are critical for the one follicle destined to become the dominant one, and in the end produce and release an egg at ovulation. The dominant follicle uses estrogen up-regulation to increase its own receptors and shut down the receptors of the other follicles it is competing with. This rather complicated process allows a woman to conceive only one child per pregnancy – for the most part.

Although required for follicle development, the up-regulation abilities of estrogen can cause major problems within the systems of the body. Most hormones attach to a receptor, do their thing, are released and escorted out of the cell. Estrogen alone can attach, release, attach again and repeat this cycle over and over again. As well, estrogen can increase the number of its own receptors, a process called replenishment Only one hormone can block the recycling of estrogen, replenishment of estrogen receptors and improve the ability of the cell to get rid of estrogen. That hormone is progesterone, which gives progesterone a special place among the sex hormones and deserves more discussion.

PROGESTERONE

The story of progesterone production follows a completely different course and it is very relevant to BHRT. In fact, the concept of estrogen/progesterone (E/P) balance is critical and one of the key areas of patient treatment. Think of progesterone as the natural balancing agent to estrogen and part of nature's safety system.

However, although progesterone can block estrogen replenishment and increase the cells' abilities to remove estrogen, progesterone production doesn't follow the same path as estrogen, which creates mismatch and sometimes adverse symptoms. The problem is that progesterone production peaks in the mid-20s and then gradually falls to very low levels during menopause. This is well-illustrated in the chart.

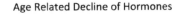

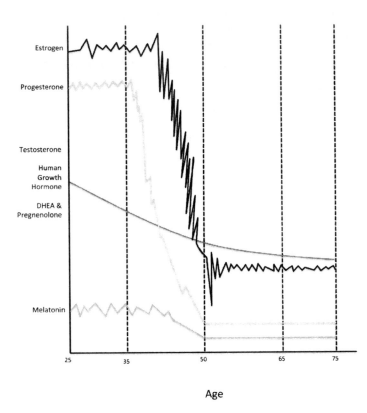

Fig. 3-2 Hormone-production decline over age

And of course, as progesterone falls and estrogen levels remain high, women may develop an increased E/P ratio. This problem can actually be worsened by lifestyle factors that increase the relative amounts of estrogen in the body. The two main culprits are weight gain and environmental exposure to phthalates. Pthalates are substances used in plastics and which contain a gas that, when absorbed into the body, mimics estrogen. (This condition of estrogen dominance was outlined by Dr. John Lee and Virginia Hopkins in their 1996 book,

What Your Doctor May Not Tell You About Menopause: The Breakthrough Book on Natural Progesterone.)

Toxic exposure to phthalates can cause estrogen dominance, which causes many of the symptoms seen by women in their 40s and early 50s. And it's important enough to deserve a chapter later in the book. Symptoms – and their severity – can be used as a guide to hormone imbalances, with measured levels as confirmation.

That's why it's important to have a good relationship with your doctor and that he/she listens. I'll also share other strategies to help you figure out what you need to know and how to interpret the information you'll receive along the way.

But I want you to know something that may make you feel better now: If you've been suffering from any of the symptoms or problems already described or to be mentioned in upcoming chapters, and imbalances are detected, interventions to restore balance are very effective for symptom relief.

If you are overweight – even just by five to 10 pounds – you are significantly more at risk of degenerative diseases such as:

- *Cancer*
- *Diabetes (type 2)*
- *Heart disease*
- *Hypertension*
- *Osteoarthritis*
- *Stroke*

If you are approximately 20% above your optimal weight, you triple your risk of having diabetes and/or high blood pressure. You also double your risk of having high cholesterol (I'll explain more in other chapters why this is dangerous and even be life-threatening), and increases your chances of having heart disease by 60%.

While you can control your weight, you can't always control your environment – and most people are shocked when they discover just how toxic their everyday environment can be. In this case, I'm talking about exposure to phthalates, substances that are added to plastics to increase their durability, longevity, flexibility and transparency. Phthalates are primarily used to soften polyvinyl chloride. They contain a gas that, once absorbed into the body, attaches to hormone receptors – because their chemical structure mimics estrogen – and damages them.

Did you know that there is so much plastic in the food supply that the U.S. government created a guideline to establish a safe daily amount that can be ingested? But they're not found only in food. They're in the water we drink and use, in our homes, our offices, even in our cars. (That new-car smell so many of us love? It comes from the phthalates escaping from a plastic dashboard after it has sat in the sun for a few days.)

And even though they are finally being phased out of many products in the European Union and the United States because of health concerns, they're still found in:

- *Enteric coatings on pills and some nutritional products*
- *Perfume*
- *Eye shadow*
- *Nail polish*

- *Moisturizers*
- *Children's toys*
- *Modeling clay*
- *Paint and paint pigments*
- *Packaging materials*
- *Shower curtains*
- *Plastic dishes*
- *Lubricants*
- *Floor tiles*
- *Emulsifying agents*
- *Suspending agents*
- *Adhesives and glues*
- *Agricultural pesticides*
- *Building materials*
- *Wrappers for food*
- *Medical devices*
- *Toothpaste*
- *Detergents*
- *Waxes*
- *Printing ink*
- *Sex toys made of "jelly rubber"*
- *Vinyl upholstery*
- *Food containers*

As of 2004, manufacturers produced about 363,000 metric tons (800 million pounds or 400,000 short tons) of phthalates each year. They contribute 10%-60% of plastic products by weight.

TESTOSTERONE

As progesterone levels start falling after about age 25, so does the body's natural testosterone production. In general, women and men alike have their highest levels of testosterone secretion in their mid-20s and then experience a gradual decline. In fact, testosterone production falls by 50% in women from age 20 to 40 and continues to fall until menopause.

After the menopausal transition, testosterone is maintained at a low and stable level for the rest of a woman's life. Production of testosterone at this point comes from the post-menopausal ovaries and the adrenal glands. Further complicating the picture is the fact that each term pregnancy is accompanied by a 10%-15% drop in testosterone production – which does not recover.

Testosterone is needed for libido, mood preservation and energy in women. It has been greatly overlooked by gynecology over the last 50 years, but in the last decade there has been increased interest. Many of the symptoms of testosterone deficiency mimic those of depression.

I truly believe that it has become acceptable, and in fact preferable, among the medical establishment to treat testosterone deficiency with antidepressants. We have an absolute plethora of antidepressant options, with new ones coming to market on a regular basis. If, in fact, antidepressants are now the preferred treatment for hormone imbalances, we have truly reached a sad state of affairs. While treatment of hormone imbalance may be good for the sales of these antidepressants, we really don't know the long-term implications of their use over many years.

Why not correct hormone imbalances with correctly prescribed hormones identical on a structural level to the hormones that are out of balance? This question may seem simple on the surface, but the implications go far deeper. Some recent studies suggest more than 20% of women ages 30 to 50 take some form of antidepressant.

Why do we have, at this time in history, a tidal wave of mood disorders? Could it be that lifestyle and environmental factors are conspiring to exacerbate hormone imbalances and deficiencies? I think so!

REAL WOMEN, REAL STORIES

Shauna

Every day, I got up with a headache and what felt like the flu. Lethargic and in pain, some days I would vomit.

It would take me several hours to feel normal enough to be able to take some form of medication to relieve the headache and be able to eat something so that I could exercise and rally enough energy to get on with the day.

As a highly functioning, 48-year-old woman, I regularly brought in a six-figure income. I was becoming increasingly unable to rely on myself to handle negotiating legal contracts and to depend on my memory in my workday.

My mind had become increasingly fuzzy. I depended on a calculator for even the simplest of calculations, then checked and double-checked everything as mistakes had become ever more common in my daily work.

My confidence was eroding as I couldn't even be sure that I would remember the names of people I saw on a regular basis. By the following year, at the age of 49, following lunch, all I wanted to do was lie down. Many days, I would do just that. Although I was exhausted, I could rarely sleep. I would remain exhausted for the rest of the day.

My annual visits to my GP always ended the same way. I would complain about all of these symptoms, he would run many tests, and pronounce me to be within the norm in all areas. He would check my FSH and announce that I wasn't in menopause. (Since I had had regular periods since the age of 12, and except for pregnancy interruptions, continued to do so, I already knew that I wasn't likely in menopause.) I believe that many people, including my GP, and possibly members of my family, thought that the problems were all in my head! One person commented that I was nearly 50! (As though I should be prepared to settle for feeling ill everyday and exhausted all the time because I was nearly 50.)

Out of desperation, I began to read about the possible causes and cures for complaints such as mine. As I had been a long- time migraine sufferer, I knew that I needed to be very careful about being prescribed estrogen, so a one-size-fits-all hormone program that combined estrogen, progesterone and testosterone was not a good choice for me.

I knew that my brother-in-law, a pharmacist, was working with a local gynecologist doing a lot of customized hormone treatments. I begged my brother-in-law for advice. He immediately referred me to Dr. Ron Brown.

Dr. Brown required a comprehensive group of tests, including blood tests to determine individual hormone levels, as well as saliva testing, done at a certain point in the cycle, and throughout the day to determine exact hormone levels.

He also required completion of an extensive questionnaire and did a personal interview to clarify the answers. He clearly understood that my issues were different from those of other patients and that he would be using my combined results to customize a treatment for me. This included thyroid medication because, as Dr. Brown pointed out, my blood tests were within the norm, but the conversion rates seemed a bit low. He also prescribed progesterone, as well as DHEA. I also started to take a good multivitamin, Vitamin D, magnesium and omega-3 capsules daily upon the advice of Dr. Brown.

Three weeks passed, and I still felt very tired. I was beginning to notice that my mental fog was lifting and that my mind was clearer, sharper, and that I felt less cranky in general.

Upon returning to be rechecked by Dr. Brown, I gave him my feedback. He increased my progesterone to 200 mg. daily. Within two more weeks, I noticed I was sleeping much more soundly, having far fewer migraine headaches, waking with a clear mind and no nausea or headache, and that I no longer felt exhausted all day long! I was stunned! My cat is now the sole occupant of my sofa during the afternoon!

I am so grateful for the persistence and patience shown by Dr. Brown in matters that so profoundly affect people's quality of life. I am forever in his debt for helping me to regain mine!

Important Points

1. Hormone production peaks at age 25 and declines for the rest of our life.

2. Individual hormones decline at different rates. This can create hormone imbalances.

3. Estrogen declines at a slower rate than progesterone and testosterone. This leads to estrogen dominance.

4. Estrogen production is increased by obesity and phthalate exposure from plastics.

5. Estrogen dominance makes weight gain easier.

6. Lack of progesterone to balance estrogen leads to heavy periods, PMS, weight gain, breast tenderness, anxiety and insomnia.

7. Low testosterone relative to estrogen leads to depression, low libido and fatigue.

8. Antidepressants are commonly used today to treat symptoms of low testosterone.

HORMONES, PATENTS AND THE PHARMACEUTICAL INDUSTRY

IS THERE A BIG CONSPIRACY?

You may be wondering what this subject has to do with the topic of BHRT. In some ways, nothing, and in some ways, everything. But it's important to go into more detail about what the pharmaceutical industry and patents have to do with this field of health – because once you do, the rest of the puzzle will fall into place, and you'll understand why the landscape looks like it does at this time.

Most modern medicines, in large part, have been developed by the major pharmaceutical companies over the last 50 years or so. The companies have funded more than 90% of the medical research, and that research has led to the development of so many life-saving remedies

So why does the established pharmaceutical industry seem to be at odds with BHRT? And why is it trying so hard to have this entire area of medicine and treatment discredited or made illegal? And is there really a conspiracy?

Certainly, there is misunderstanding and even a lack of reason in both camps – and this has slowed progress on the health promotion front – but I really don't believe there are any bad guys on the scene.

SHOW THEM THE MONEY

First of all, pharmaceutical companies are primarily in business to make a profit – and there's nothing wrong with that. Like other public corporations, pharmaceutical companies have a responsibility to their shareholders and strive to produce a profit.

Medical research – and drug development in particular – is a very costly and resource-dependent endeavor.

It takes millions of dollars and many years to move a drug from conception through research and development to clinical trials and all the way to being approved and sold on the market. In fact, only a handful of drugs that start this process manage to hit the pharmacy shelf.

Some products make it partway through only to run into a problem and never reach the market. The costs of these failures must be covered by the drugs that do make it. In the long run, pharmaceutical companies have developed thousands of drugs that have dramatically improved the human experience.

The patent process was developed to help pharmaceutical companies cover the cost of drug development. Without patents, there would be no financial incentive to develop new drugs – and that part of the system would collapse. A patent permits the company to sell a particular drug that it has developed without competition from other companies for a specified number of years. This allows the company to recoup its research and development costs.

Once a drug patent has expired, competitors can produce generic products without the same R&D costs, which lowers the cost to patients. In fact, there are some generic drug companies whose only function is to produce generic copies of name-brand drugs when the patent expires.

All pharmaceutical companies are in the search for so-called blockbuster drugs, ones that treat a problem or symptom that is common in the population. Recent blockbusters include Lipitor (high cholesterol), Viagra (erectile dysfunction) and Prozac (depression). These drugs changed the treatment of a common disease and received a commanding percentage of the market for that medical problem.

Blockbusters create large profits for the company lucky or talented enough to invent or discover the drug and those profits allow the whole cycle to start again. This is the base of our capitalistic system. It also, in part, is the driving force for the rapid pace of medical treatment advancement.

The problem is, the benefits of this process are also the Achilles heel of the system.

A drug that could cure a particular disease in a short period of time would be unlikely to generate sufficient profits to cover its R&D costs. Instead, the ideal drug would be one that could control the symptoms of a common medical condition – without curing the underlying condition. This would allow the company with the patent an opportunity to recoup its expenses for product development. And since more than 90% of medical research is pharmaceutically sponsored, this has led to a less-than-optimal situation.

Research is now directed toward studies that either expand indications for an existing drug, or find new uses for a drug the company already produces, drugs that control symptoms, rather than for a cure for a particular disease.

So, knowing the way the system is set up, is it any surprise that cures for our common diseases seem elusive at best? Conspiracy theorists would say the cures exist but never see the light of day. I do not believe their arguments, but do feel that the present situation does not serve the public interest as well as it could.

PATENT LAW AND BHRT

One of the basic elements of drug patent law is that a company can't patent a naturally occurring compound. These include estrogen, testosterone, progesterone and DHEA. If a company can't obtain a patent, why would it sponsor and fund research on compounds that will never provide sufficient profits to generate a reasonable return after expenses?

The only option to a pharmaceutical company interested in the area of hormone replacement is to develop a hormone analogue (a compound with a molecular structure closely similar to that of another). This involves modifying the native hormone – for example progesterone – and finding a synthetic compound that acts like progesterone in the body. If such a compound can be developed, it can be patented and sold at a profit. This is the situation with medroxyprogesterone acetate, or Provera, an analogue of progesterone. Since Provera is not progesterone, it is called a progestin, and the distinction between progesterone and a progestin can't be overemphasized – which is why we'll be going over it in a later chapter.

When Provera was first developed, it was the only way to give a woman progesterone, as there was no natural progesterone product available. The development of Provera was critical, as it is necessary to prevent uterine cancer in women undergoing estrogen replacement therapy for menopausal symptoms.

Luckily, since then, natural progesterone products have been developed to avoid some of the problems seen with progestin therapy. Unfortunately, life is not always simple and so it was with Provera and the other progestins.

We've already discussed the concept of hormone-receptor interaction as being similar to a key-in-the-lock process. It turns out that even small changes to the structure of a natural hormone – so that it can be patented – creates subtle changes in the action of that analogue in the body. An altered hormone may over- or under-stimulate its own receptor, or bind to a receptor of a different hormone and create unexpected or unwanted effects.

The chart below shows the difference between progesterone and Provera, the chemical change to the progesterone molecule allowed a patent to be granted for Provera. The chart also shows how small changes to a hormone molecule can have dramatic changes in function. The structural difference between progesterone and testosterone is very small, and yet they function in the body in dramatically different ways. So doesn't it seem simplistic to believe that the alterations of progesterone to form Provera may not have unintended consequences?

Understanding Hormone Composition

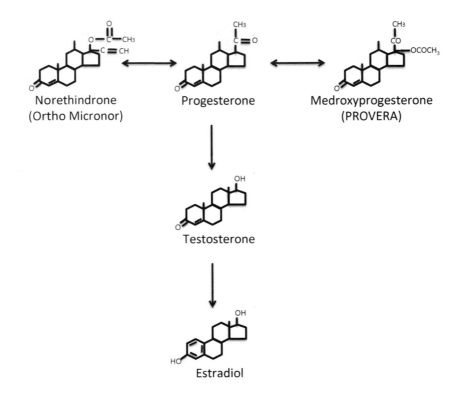

Fig. 4-1: Hormone composition

As we can see, all steroid hormones, natural and synthetic, are not equal. Perhaps the wisdom of the body and evolution have been able to work things out better, with respect to safety and function, than we can in our laboratories.

Bioidentical hormones are identical to natural human hormones on a molecular level. As a result, they can't be granted a patent. But the very system that provides a degree of safety prevents further funded research into their use – because there's just no potential for extraordinary profit – and no reason for any pharmaceutical company to spend money on BHRT.

There are no bad guys here, just two different camps with different realities, goals and points of view. The rest of this book will explain why there are some significant advantages to BHRT and why the government – the agent of the people – needs to step up with funding. Research is urgently needed to confirm safety and prove that BHRT is an effective and cost-efficient approach to health promotion in the 21st century.

Important Points

1. Pharmaceutical companies and the research they generate are responsible for many of the advances in medical care over the last 50 years.

2. Medication research, development and clinical trials are very expensive and necessary for public safety.

3. Pharmaceutical companies answer to shareholders and require profits to survive.

4. The patent process was developed to help companies cover drug-development costs and encourage research.

5. Drug development is directed toward agents that control the symptoms of common diseases. This has directed medical research away from methods that cure or prevent diseases.

6. There is no profit in the cure of diseases.

7. Patents cannot be granted for a naturally occurring substance or hormone.

8. A hormone must be modified on a chemical basis to be granted a patent.

9. Small changes to hormone structure can result in significant changes in the resulting hormone function.

10. There are few opportunities for patents in the agents used for BHRT. This limits the profit potential for BHRT.

11. No profit potential means limited availability for research funding for BHRT.

12. Government funding is urgently needed to allow research into the effectiveness and safety of BHRT.

CHAPTER 5

THE WOMEN'S HEALTH INITIATIVE

You may be wondering why there is any reluctance from women or the medical profession to consider HRT – especially since the advantages of using it are so overwhelming, including a dramatic and lasting improvement in the quality of life during menopause.

But the sad truth is, although many women have one or more often debilitating symptoms, they are afraid – in some cases, even terrified – to go on hormone therapy. In fact, only about 30% of prescriptions written for HRT are ever filled.

Gynecologists have seen the benefits of HRT, and numerous studies have proven its worth. In fact, the Society of Obstetricians and Gynecologists of Canada is sponsoring a series of public forums across Canada to try to dispel some of the myths about HRT.

To understand where the problem comes from, we have to look at the history of hormone replacement therapy.

A QUICK TRIP DOWN MEMORY LANE

When Ayerst, McKenna and Harrison Pharmaceutical Corp. merged with American Home Products to became Wyeth Pharmaceutical Corp., and introduced Premarin in 1942, it brought sudden relief of menopausal symptoms to hundreds of thousands of women.

Premarin was created by extracting estrogen from the concentrated urine of pregnant mares – which is also how it got its name: **PRE**gnant **MAR**es' ur**INE**. And it's still created the same way – thousands upon thousands of pregnant mares are held in stalls, with funnels attached to collect the highly concentrated urine. The conditions the mares must endure caused concern among animal-rights activists.

Premarin was prescribed to women with symptoms of estrogen deficiency in an unopposed fashion; that is, they were given just Premarin, whether they had a uterus or not. It didn't seem as if much thought or concern had been given to long-term consequences. However, it was eventually revealed in the mid-'60s that not only had there been concern, but some quiet studies proved there was an increased risk of endometrial cancer (cancer of the lining of the uterus) connected to the use of unopposed Premarin in women who had not had a hysterectomy.

This, of course, resulted in a backlash among women who avoided HRT because of this increased risk.

Premarin was one of Wyeth's biggest sellers. So, with women suddenly terrified of taking this drug, something had to be done. Research in the 1970s found that the use of a progesterone-like drug called Provera at a dose of 10 mg for 12-14 days of each month would prevent the development of uterine cancer in women taking Premarin.

However, it had one undesirable effect in the eyes of the women who were taking it: They would continue to have menstrual cycles, or resume them if menopausal, for as long as they were on the medication. This put post-menopausal women with a uterus, suffering from estrogen deficiency, between a rock and a hard place. The only benefit of menopause was the loss of periods, but the treatment of symptoms meant the resumption of periods. And so the drug companies went back to the drawing board and began to look for new treatment ideas and methods.

Additional testing in the 1980s found that Provera, given in low doses every day instead of the 12-14-day interval, would prevent regular menstruation when used with Premarin. At last, it seemed as if researchers had found the ideal situation. With this regime, a woman could enjoy all the benefits of estrogen therapy and none of the disadvantages of regular menstrual cycles.

MENOPAUSE AND THE INCREASED RISK OF HEART DISEASE

At that same time, evidence had been accumulating that estrogen therapy in postmenopausal women seemed to decrease the incidence of heart disease. This was important, because heart disease in women increases dramatically after menopause. Data from the U.S. National Vital Statistic Report show that death rates from heart disease double in women between ages 45-55 and 55-64 years[1]. Even more alarming is the 12-fold increase in heart disease death rates from ages 55-64 and ages 75-84.

Numerous animal and human studies showed estrogen had a protective effect against development of heart disease. Since heart disease becomes the major killer of women after menopause, these findings appeared to be very important.

Through HRT, not only could women avoid the ravages of estrogen-deficiency symptoms, they could also reduce the incidence of heart disease. Add to this the newly developing regime of continuous combined estrogen and progestin, it seemed to be an ideal situation. Thrown into the mix was the suggestion that estrogen replacement seemed to decrease the chances of developing osteoporosis, bowel cancer and Alzheimer's disease, and all seemed to be well.

The only thing that was needed was proof of this benefit, and medicine had the means to significantly improve the lot of women the world over. The most powerful of study designs is the double-blinded, randomized placebo-controlled trial. In this type of trial, neither the patient nor investigators know whether the patient is on the study drug or a placebo. A placebo has no drug activity and is used to compare the treatment being investigated with no treatment at all. This study design removes many sources of potential bias and is considered the gold standard of investigations.

And thus began the Women's Health Initiative, or WHI.[2]

Funded by Wyeth Pharmaceuticals in conjunction with the National Institutes of Health, this was the largest study ever put together in women's health. There were two arms in the WHI study, which were determined by whether the participants had undergone a hysterectomy.

Participants who had not had a hysterectomy were placed into the continuous, combined estrogen/progestin arm of the study. This was to prevent development of uterine cancer with the use of unopposed estrogen seen in post-menopausal women with a uterus. Women who had undergone a hysterectomy were placed into the unopposed-estrogen arm of the study, as they were not considered at risk of uterine cancer. They were instructed to take Premarin daily without Provera.

The aim of the study was to conclusively demonstrate that the use of HRT in asymptomatic, post-menopausal women prevented fatal heart disease and improved the quality of life for women. Make sure you note that the women enrolled were asymptomatic ie: they didn't suffer from hot flashes. It was already established that symptomatic women could take Premarin with or without Provera. If successful, this study would have been very significant evidence to support the use of these particular medicines in post-menopausal women. And this of course, would have been very financially rewarding to Wyeth and was the reason it funded the study.

THE FIRST ARM OF THE STUDY

In the continuous, combined arm of the study, for women with no prior hysterectomy, participants were given (in a randomized, blinded fashion), Premarin .625 mg and Provera 2.5 mg per day (combined in a capsule and called Prempro) or placebo.

Neither the investigators nor the patients knew what medicine was being used for a particular woman.

In all, 16,608 post-menopausal women with no previous hysterectomy were enrolled from 1993 to 1998 at 40 clinical centers. The women were between 50-79 years old, and were excluded if they had had breast cancer or a medical condition likely to result in death within three years.

After a mean follow-up of 5.2 years, the WHI safety monitoring board recommended the immediate discontinuation of the study due to an increased risk of breast cancer in women on Prempro. In this treated group of women, there was a 24% increase in the diagnosis of breast cancer.

Also, breast density on mammography increased in the women on Prempro, indicating breast tissue stimulation by this hormone combination. And to make matters worse, further analysis showed this group of women had a 29% increase in coronary heart disease, a 41% increase in the risk of stroke, and a 110% increase in the risk of blood clots and pulmonary emboli.

I still remember the day the study was terminated and the media was alerted to the results. The phone lines to our OB/GYN practice were flooded with concerned women asking for direction regarding their HRT. As a group of gynecologists, we had not bought into the concept of treating asymptomatic women with hormones to prevent disease. Our patients on HRT were being treated for symptoms of menopause and the study results had little effect on our practice. But it was still unsettling.

THE SECOND ARM OF THE STUDY

The second arm of the study was with women who had had a hysterectomy; 9,739 of them with an average age of 63 were enrolled into the estrogen-only arm of the study. Without a uterus, these women were treated only with daily Premarin .625 mg per day or placebo.

Gynecology has for many years had a motto: "No uterus – no progesterone." (I'll have much more to say about this.) Even after the first arm of the study was stopped, this arm was allowed to continue, as there was no increased risk of breast cancer seen in this group.

Unfortunately, in 2004, this arm of the study was prematurely stopped due to a 40% increase in the risk of stroke and a 34% increase in the risk of blood clots. I say unfortunately because this group of women showed a 10% decrease in heart disease and a 23% decrease in the risk of breast cancer.

The reduction in the risk of breast cancer was the most surprising, as OB/GYNs had always thought that estrogen therapy increased the risk of breast cancer. The results of both arms are shown in the table below. They are shown as an odds ratio (OR). If the risk is equal to placebo, the OR is 1.00. A number above 1.00 indicates an increased risk and vice versa.

	Arm1 CEE/MPA	Arm 2 CEE
Number	16,608	9,739
Mean Age	63	63
Coronary Heart Disease	1.29	0.91
Breast Cancer	1.26	0.77
Stroke	1.41	1.39
Blood Clots/Emboli	2.13	1.34

In both groups, there was a small reduction in the risk of hip fracture and colon cancer. However, neither of these benefits was large enough to balance the increased risk of breast cancer in the Prempro group, or the increased risk of stroke and blood clots in the Premarin-only arm.

After the dust settled and numerous analyses were done, a few important conclusions were reached – and a few were overlooked.

THE REST OF THE STORY

The study failed to show that HRT using an oral estrogen with progestin was a health-promoting intervention in asymptomatic, post-menopausal women. That is why it's also important to point out some of the major shortcomings of the WHI study.

For example, the group of women in the study had an average age of 63 – which means they were long past menopause, which on average starts at age 51. And remember, the incidence of heart disease accelerates in women after menopause.

One of the biggest problems with the entire study was that an EKG was used to screen for existing heart disease. Today, we know EKG simply is not specific or sensitive enough to pick up existing heart disease or coronary vessel blockage. That meant many women enrolled in the study already had asymptomatic coronary heart disease. And we also know from previous studies that hormone treatments do not reduce the rate of heart attacks in women with existing heart disease.

The HERS (Heart and Estrogen/Progestin Replacement Study) trial of the 1990s looked at the effect of estrogen and progestin treatment in women who had already had a heart attack. It found that HRT in women with a previous coronary event did not reduce the risk of subsequent heart attacks[3]. Indeed, in the first year of treatment, these women showed an increase in the risk of another heart attack. Therefore, if poor patient screening allowed the inclusion of a large number of women with existing coronary vessel disease, we would expect this to reduce the effectiveness of any HRT effect. But it's important to note that much of the observed increase in heart disease and stroke was directly attributable to the poor patient selection of the WHI.

In general, many women will become symptomatic and go on HRT during peri-menopause or early menopause, (i.e. between the ages of 45-55). These women have a much lower intrinsic risk of already having heart disease, which does not respond to HRT. We would expect this younger group of women to experience the cardio-protective benefits of HRT that have been demonstrated in many animal and human trials.

Also, newer research indicates that Provera, when used continuously, is able to offset the heart benefits of estrogen. I will have more to say on this in a future chapter.

The second major failing of the WHI study was the unfortunate choice of an oral, or pill, form of estrogen. Because, again, today we know that oral estrogen increases the liver's production of clotting proteins. And so both arms of the study saw an increase in the risk of blood clots, pulmonary emboli and stroke.

Now we know that transdermal administration of estrogen, using patches and creams, does not increase the risk of these unpredictable and occasionally fatal events. But Wyeth did not have a transdermal preparation at the time, and one of its goals was probably to increase the sales of its flagship estrogen product, Premarin.

I believe the third and biggest mistake of the WHI was its selection of Provera as the progestational agent to prevent endometrial hyperplasia, a precursor to uterine cancer, and cancer of the uterus.

In 1995, the Postmenopausal Estrogen/Progestin Interventions (PEPI) trial clearly demonstrated that cyclic micronized progesterone, which is an oral form of natural or bioidentical progesterone, had a more favourable effect on cholesterol and fibrinogen levels than either cyclic or continuous Provera[4].

And in 1999, Dr. Thomas Clarkson reported that medroxyprogesterone acetate MPA, or Provera, directly opposes many of the beneficial effects of estrogen on the heart and blood vessels[5] Further, he showed that MPA reduces the dilation effect of estrogen on the coronary arteries, and it was associated with an increase in insulin resistance, progression of coronary atherosclerosis, and acceleration of low-density lipoprotein (LDL) uptake into plaque lesions of the vessels.

All in all, MPA, or Provera, is not a good choice for reducing the risk of heart disease and stroke. It seems to directly oppose the beneficial effects of estrogen on the heart when it is used on a daily basis. MPA is safe when used for 12-14 days out of the month, but most women will not accept the benefits of HRT if they have to continue their periods into the menopause Natural progesterone in pill or cream form, does not oppose the favorable actions of estrogen and should be the agent of choice for HRT. Pill, or oral, forms of estrogen increase the risks of blood clots and strokes, and should not be used. Transdermal or cream forms of estrogen are effective and much safer.

THE AFTERMATH

The backlash to the WHI has been truly horrendous. HRT was cast as a cancer promoter, probably one of the worst of all women's fears. Even today, we're still fighting the adverse effects of this study on women's perceptions.

The media must also bear some of the responsibility for the continued problem, because in the scramble to capitalize on all the drama and headlines, they missed some of the important points I've just shared with you. Sadly, once the media furor had subsided, little attempt was made to educate the public about the very real and provable shortcomings of the study.

The most interesting aspect to this whole sad story is the lack of attention paid to estrogen and breast cancer. We have for many years believed that estrogen increased the risk of breast cancer. But in the WHI, the estrogen-only group had a 23% decrease in breast cancer diagnosis. No mention of this was ever made by the researchers, reviewers or the media, even though the cumulative difference in breast cancer risk between the two treatment groups approached 50%.

It would appear that oral Premarin alone decreases the risk of breast cancer. Continuous use of Provera seems to dramatically increase the risk of breast cancer. I still know of many doctors prescribing continuous Provera to their patients on HRT despite this strong data. Cyclic Provera doesn't increase breast cancer risk. Why has no attention been paid to the issue of breast cancer risk increases seen with continuous Provera use? I have no answer, but will NEVER have any of my patients use Provera on a continuous basis!

HRT was labeled as the villain, and women were left to fend for themselves with the ravages caused by the symptoms of menopause.

Over time, the medical community has come to understand the study's flaws, but an entire generation of women was led to believe that all hormones increase the risk of cancer. As I hope you're beginning to see, however – and as I will continue to attempt to prove – nothing could be further from the truth.

Important Points

1. Estrogen-replacement therapy dramatically reduces the symptoms of estrogen deficiency seen in women as they go through the menopausal transition.

2. Estrogen should be given transdermally (cream) to reduce the risks of stroke and blood clots.

3. Premarin was the first estrogen developed and was quite effective in treating those symptoms. Use of Premarin alone in a woman with a uterus, however, increases her risk of uterine cancer

4. Addition of a progestin, such as Provera, for 12-14 days of each month prevents the increased risk of uterine cancer seen with the use of unopposed estrogen. Unfortunately, cyclic Provera means continuation of regular periods as long as the treatment is used.

5. Provera, when used every day of the cycle, appears to reverse the benefits of estrogen in prevention of heart disease.

6. Provera used in a continuous fashion also seems to increase the risk of breast cancer.

7. Natural progesterone doesn't interfere with the beneficial effects of estrogen on heart disease prevention.

8. Natural progesterone doesn't increase the risk of breast cancer when used in a continuous fashion with estrogen

9. Estrogen and natural progesterone should always be used together, whether or not a woman has had a hysterectomy.

1 Statistics, NCFH. Deaths, percent of total deaths, and death rates for the 10 leading causes of death in selected age groups, by race and sex; United States, 2000-Con. National Vital Statistics report 2002; 50:1-85 / 2 The Women's Health Initiative Study Group. Control Clin Trials 1998; 19; 61-109 / 3 Heart and Estrogen/progesterone Replacement Study JAMA, 1998, 280: 605-13 / 4 The postmenopausal Estrogen/Progestin (PEPI) Trial JAMA 1995, vol 273, no.3; 199-208 5 Jour Repro Med 1999, vol44, no.2; 180-184.

CHAPTER 6

WHAT ESTROGEN DOMINANCE MEANS TO YOU

Hormones continually change from the time a woman starts to menstruate until menopause. Even after menopause, hormone levels are in a constant state of flux. It has taken many years from the discovery of hormones to reach today's appreciation of their balance to each other.

As I've stated earlier, the absolute levels of hormones **are not as important** as the balance of each hormone with its natural partners. There is no better example than the balance of estrogen and progesterone.

To recap, hormone production peaks for most of us around age 25. For women, from there until menopause, estrogen secretion is relatively stable and does not fall much. Close to menopause, estrogen production starts to fluctuate with large up-and-down swings until it finally falls dramatically with menopause. It is only when a woman has gone 12 months without a period that doctors can even confidently say that she has entered menopause.

However, the picture is quite different for progesterone. Its production peaks in the mid-20s and then steadily falls for the next 25 years or so. Levels drop by 50% by about the age of 40, and they continue to decline until menopause.

Since progesterone is the natural balance or antagonist to estrogen, this sets up a very significant imbalance. Additional factors contribute to this imbalance and create estrogen dominance, a phrase coined by Dr. John Lee that refers to the common imbalance of progesterone to estrogen. In *What Your Doctor May Not Tell You About Menopause: The Breakthrough Book on Natural Progesterone*, he and coauthor Virginia Hopkins broke ground in the importance of this hormone balance for women.

Even a small degree of estrogen dominance sets up a disturbance in thyroid hormone function. This is significant, because the thyroid hormone establishes our metabolic rate and ability to burn calories. Excess estrogen increases the thyroid-binding proteins in the blood – which means the amount of free thyroid hormone that keeps your metabolism going is also reduced. Reduced metabolic rate leads to weight gain as the calories aren't burnt as fast as they are taken in.

Almost any degree of estrogen dominance seems to contribute to easy weight gain. This could be aggravated by the antagonism of insulin creating a degree of insulin resistance, as well as the interference in thyroid function. Insulin resistance leads to the need for higher levels of insulin to expedite movement of blood glucose into muscle, nerve and fat cells for metabolism. High insulin levels contribute to extra storage of glucose in fat cells, and resultant weight gain. Low thyroid function and insulin resistance create conditions for easy weight gain.

Unfortunately as women gain weight, their metabolism down-shifts, starting a vicious cycle. Fat tissue is not just those unsightly bulges that we hate to see. It is metabolically very active and produces its own hormones – and guess what? It can cause a further imbalance to the hormone harmony in the body. Fat cells are able to convert an adrenal hormone called androstenedione into a weak estrogen, estrone. And because the adrenal glands are always busy producing androstenedione, there is never a shortage of estrogen-precursor hormone.

And that's where the vicious cycle comes in – weight gain in women and men causes estrogen dominance in the body, which brings a tendency to gain even more weight. But then, to top things off, changes in our environment over the last 50 years have added to the problem, and further upset the delicate balance within our bodies.

THE PROBLEM WITH PLASTICS AND OTHER ENVIRONMENTAL BAD GUYS

One of the biggest changes to upset the hormonal-balance applecart comes from plastic. Plastics are everywhere in our lives, and, at first glance, seemed to be an amazing convenience. Probably one of their most popular uses is for storing – and reheating – leftovers.

But here's the problem: Plastics contain large amounts of phthalates, whose chemical structures look like estrogen, so much so, in fact, that they and the many compounds like them have been called xenoestrogens. Xenestrogens mimic estrogens in the body and contribute to estrogen dominance.

When plastic gets hot – such as when leftovers are microwaved – they release even higher levels of phthalates and related compounds. The same thing happens if you drink water or other liquids from a plastic bottle that has been exposed to heat and sunlight – increased levels of xenoestrogens are released.

Unluckily, the problem doesn't stop there. Many of the pesticides and organic solvents used in our food and water supplies act as xenoestrogens, too. And we don't even know how to measure them in order to get an idea of the overall levels of xenoestrogens in the environment.

So as you can see, many factors contribute to the development of estrogen dominance. In fact, it is the single most common problem I see in women before the age of 50. The imbalances wreak havoc and may affect everything from your mood to those nagging little aches and pains, to your body's ability to lose weight, fight illness or infection, and the fluctuations in your energy level.

WHAT YOU NEED TO KNOW ABOUT ESTROGEN

The body produces three types of estrogen in different percentages and uses each one as needed. Estrone is a weak estrogen primarily produced by conversion of androstenedione in fat tissue. Obesity increases the production of estrone even in the post-menopausal woman. Estradiol is the most powerful and the primary estrogen of pre menopausal women. The third is estriol, a weak estrogen that is produced in significant quantities only in pregnancy.

Each one of the estrogens has different functions and different effects. Estradiol has been proven to prevent osteoporosis, but it may also contribute to the development of breast and uterine cancer. On the other hand, estriol may provide protection against breast and uterine cancers.

This is another reason that BHRT may be right for you – most BHRT treatments usually include the cancer-fighting estriol, which is not found in the pharmaceutical estrogens.

The decline in estrogen production is different in each woman, based on body mass index. For instance, estrogen production usually declines at a more rapid rate in women who are thin, but may not decline at all in women who are overweight. And because of that, women who are overweight often experience estrogen dominance.

Estrogen dominance usually occurs in overweight women when their fat tissue converts adrenally produced androstenedione to estrone (a fairly weak form of estrogen) and then indirectly to estradiol.

The "advantage," if you want to call it that, is that overweight women seldom have hot flashes during menopause. However, they are much more likely to develop endometrial cancer (the mucous membrane that lines the uterus). This is due to the low-level stimulation by estrone on the lining of the uterus over the course of many years.

Estrogen has as many as 400 crucial functions, in approximately 300 tissues of the body. Separate and widely distributed tissues such as brain, bone, ovaries, vagina, bladder, uterus, eyes, heart, blood vessels and lungs, all have estrogen receptors. Estrogen performs very important functions in these tissues and organs. Some of the vital jobs that estrogen helps with are listed below.

ESTROGEN
Increases the metabolic rate, unless there is too much estrogen
Helps to regulate body temperature
Enhances magnesium absorption
Improves insulin sensitivity
Improves arterial elasticity
Decreases platelet adhesion
Improves sleep
Prevents muscle damage
Reduces blood vessel plaque formation
Maintains muscle mass
Dilates small arteries
Decreases LDL and its oxidation which is bad for the endothelial lining
Maintains memory
Enhances mood and concentration (through production of serotonin)
Augments bone density
Stimulates the production of choline acetyltransferase (reduces risk of Alzheimer's)
Stimulates increased production of HDL (reduces risk of heart disease by 40% -50%)
Helps prevent tooth loss
Reduces risk of colon cancer
Improves sex drive

Table 6-1: Estrogen functions

With all of the critical body functions that estrogen participates in, how can estrogen dominance be a problem? Even though estrogen is critical for proper body function, like most things in life, you can get too much of a good thing! An improper balance of estrogen to progesterone can create a bewildering combination of symptoms that can literally affect the entire body. The table below lists some of the symptoms of estrogen dominance.

SYMPTOMS OF ESTROGEN DOMINANCE INCLUDE:
Anxiety
Panic attacks
Depression
Irritability
Mood swings
Insomnia
Pain
Inflammation of joints
Bloating
Heavy menstrual bleeding
Carbohydrate cravings
Sore, swollen or tender breasts
Difficulty concentrating or staying focused
Headaches/migraines before periods
Unexplained weight gain
Water retention
Frequent yeast infections
Lack of sex drive
Fibrocystic breast tissue
Uterine fibroids
Sudden feelings of "weepiness"

Table 6-2: Estrogen dominance

One of the biggest problems for women with these symptoms is that estrogen dominance is often misdiagnosed, and the usual treatment is antidepressants and other medications; or worse, the symptoms are overlooked altogether and chalked up to being part of the normal side effects of aging. A quick look at this symptom list will alarm most female readers. This list of symptoms includes a large proportion of the complaints that women present to their primary care provider. Symptoms of poor body function are the only means of communication the body has. Proper body function is the default position and shows up as a condition of "ease". Improper function is a condition of "dis" "ease", or what we call symptoms. The body is always correct when it is communicating symptoms of imbalance. It can't tell us there is too much estrogen directly. The body sends us messages in the form of symptoms, to tell us all is not well. How we interpret and react to these symptoms determines where we go from here. Lifestyle changes and treatment choices that reestablish balance allow the symptoms to disappear. Failure to recognize the imbalance and covering up of the symptoms with a pharmaceutical agent, does nothing to reestablish a condition of "ease". Covering up symptoms allows the "disease" process to continue unopposed, until the very function of that tissue is compromised.

When we consider the whole issue of estrogen-progesterone balance, we can see that more than one possibility exists for estrogen dominance. Normal estrogen with low progesterone will look identical to high estrogen and normal/low progesterone. In fact, low estrogen with even lower progesterone will still look like estrogen dominance! Testing is required to establish the basic estrogen level to determine the exact imbalance. Once you know the imbalance, treatment is relatively straightforward. Since conventional medicine doesn't recognize the concept of estrogen/progesterone balance, these practitioners are handicapped in their approach to their patient's symptoms. That's why it's so important to see a doctor who is trained in BHRT and can administer the proper tests.

I have great hopes that in the near future, there will be a convergence of the two schools of thought. We are truly in very exciting times as the general level of knowledge in the population increases as a result of the internet. This is part of the process the Ray Kurzweil and Dr. Terry Grossman alluded to in their book *Fantastic Voyage*. No longer is the average man or woman completely dependent on their health care practitioner for health advice. In fact, an interested person can learn an incredible amount about a disease process in a few hours on the "net". I believe that in the not too distant future, there will be a more collaborative approach to health care. This will take the shape of a partnership between the patient and practitioner.

The most exciting part of this is well seen in the whole area of bio-identical hormones. Since there is no support in conventional medicine for this area, why is it expanding so rapidly? Just as that "irritating" patient raised a question with me that led me to these concepts, more and more patients will influence their practitioners. However, there are forces at work even beyond those already discussed. Bio-identical hormones have received much publicity from celebrities such as Oprah, Dr. Oz and Robin McGraw. Certainly, the most outspoken and visible proponent of BHRT in recent years has been Suzanne Somers. Suzanne has written a number of books on this whole area of health with a focus on alternative approaches to common health problems. BHRT is one of the areas she has written about in her book *Ageless: The Naked Truth About Bioidentical Hormones*. This book is an excellent read and one of the main reasons behind this book. Many of my patients are confused about the issues of hormones and cancer, as well as the differences between pharmaceutical and bioidentical hormones. While the information in Suzanne's book is accurate, I do not agree with all of her recommendations. Also, from an academic medical point of view, it is uncomfortable to refer patients to a celebrity book in their quest for information. This discomfort eventually led to the need to write a book of information from a medical point of view, with references included to give the average person more comfort in the science behind BHRT. And here we are!

CONVENTIONAL MEDICAL BELIEFS
ABOUT ESTROGEN DOMINANCE

I have seen literally hundreds of women in the last two years whom I recognized as experiencing the symptoms of estrogen dominance. Before then, I was a conventional gynecologist who was never taught about – and did not believe in – estrogen dominance, I never saw a patient with this problem. This disconnect illustrates one of the main problems here. We will never "see" what we can't recognize.

To a conventional gynecologist, there is no such thing as estrogen/progesterone balance. In fact, conventional teaching says the only purpose for progesterone is to prevent estrogen from going wild and producing uterine cancer. A well-established dictum in gynecology says, "No uterus, no progesterone," when it comes to post-menopausal hormone replacement. There has never been a discussion of estrogen/progesterone balance in gynecology, except in the context of anovulation (the lack of regular periods).

After the egg is released in ovulation, the corpus luteum (what is left of the follicle after a woman ovulates) produces 10 days of progesterone to mature the lining of the uterus to get it ready to accept a fertilized egg. If a woman fails to produce an egg on a monthly basis, the lining of the uterus doesn't mature, and heavy, irregular menstrual bleeding will occur. This is called anovulatory dysfunctional uterine bleeding. I know it is a mouthful, but all it really says is that there is abnormal, unpredictable and often heavy menstrual bleeding as a result of sporadic or absent ovulation.

In such cases, gynecologists often use cyclic progestin therapy to induce regular periods and control heavy, irregular bleeding. I have not found natural progesterone (in either cream or pill form) to be useful in this specific situation of anovulation, and I believe cyclic progestin therapy, or the birth control pill, to be the best approach in most cases. Other corrective procedures that have been – and still are – used include D and C, endometrial ablation and hysterectomy. While these may control heavy menstruation, they do nothing to address the other symptoms of estrogen dominance.

Headaches, emotional symptoms and weight gain send the women to a family doctor, where the common treatment (after the usual blood tests show nothing wrong) is a proverbial pat on the head, and a prescription for either antidepressant, antianxiety or sleeping pills.

I can't help wondering how many thousands of women who have gone through this particular scenario have been left feeling like the real problems are all in their head? In fact, one of the biggest challenges I face every day is to teach women to believe that their symptoms are real.

Symptoms are like signposts in the fog to guide us toward balance in these very important hormones. They need to be given the attention they deserve and are more important than the simplistic tests we have available for hormone levels at this time.

Another problem is that modern medicine has become more and more time-constrained as practitioners struggle to make a reasonable living with the shrinking reimbursement payments from insurance and, in Canada, government. Doctors are forced to deal with ever-increasing rules, regulations and seemingly endless piles of red tape. And in some cases, doctors are even given specific times for the length of patient visits. Which means, in many cases, doctors have less time to spend with each patient.

Many patients have seen and felt this change – either from a negative or seemingly patronizing response from their doctor when they've given him/her a list of symptoms. Or they may have felt as if their doctor was in such a hurry that the knee-jerk reaction was to prescribe pills to treat the symptoms, rather than getting to the bottom of the cause. It's a no-win situation for everyone, which is one reason I've written this book.

Because detailed and organized symptom lists can be of assistance to you and your doctor, I've included several in later parts of this book. If you'd like to take a symptom list to your doctor, they're available for free on my website, mytruebalance.ca. Simply download the list you want, print it out and take it with you.

TYPICAL TREATMENTS FOR ESTROGEN DOMINANCE

In general, the solution to estrogen dominance are lifestyle changes in the form of diet and exercise as a prescription, and/or progesterone treatment. Many other books have written about nutrition and exercise. I will have more to say about this area in the last chapter. Suffice it to say, I believe diet and exercise are critical and often overlooked when dealing with unpleasant symptoms. Many symptoms and diseases can be cured with attention to these ares. We remain a society focused on the "pill" approach to our health and I can only trust this will change in the near future.

We have already made the distinction between a progestin and progesterone. All references to treatment are for natural progesterone. For estrogen dominance, progesterone therapy can be prescribed in either pill or cream forms. Micronized progesterone is available in a pharmaceutical preparation called Prometrium, or in a compounded micronized progesterone, which you can only get through a compounding pharmacy.

Warning: Before we go further into this section, I want to emphasize the importance of talking to your doctor if you believe you may have estrogen dominance. **DO NOT TRY TO SELF-MED-ICATE.** *I can't stress this strongly enough.*

Oral progesterone is usually prescribed in a dose of 25-200 mg daily, and, if taken 15 minutes before bed, is a very effective remedy for insomnia – a common symptom of estrogen dominance. Oral progesterone is absorbed in the small intestine, and metabolized in the liver to 5-allopregnenolone, a natural agent for sleep induction. One benefit of oral progesterone is that it cannot be converted to estrogen and testosterone by the body. *Special note: Do not take micronized progesterone before sex, as it seems to dramatically reduce the normal sexual response!* It is very bad for your partner's fragile ego to see you fall asleep during lovemaking!

Progesterone can also be used as a transdermal cream with excellent effect. I often use a combination of micronized progesterone and cream, depending on the woman's mix of symptoms. Progesterone cream at a dose of 20-80 mg/day is usually well-tolerated and can be titrated (to the lowest effective dose) by the patient to alleviate her symptoms.

Many patients increase their dose in the luteal, or pre-menstrual, phase of their cycle to combat symptoms of breast tenderness and PMS with great effect.

ESTROGEN AND UTERINE CANCER

Contrary to commonly held beliefs, transdermal progesterone can be measured in the blood and does reverse the effects of estrogen stimulation on the lining of the uterus. In our chapter on progesterone, we will look at studies proving transdermal progesterone can prevent estrogen-induced uterine (endometrial) hyperplasia and cancer. If estrogen is given without adequate progesterone, a buildup in the glandular lining of the uterus, or endometrium, can occur. This is called endometrial hyperplasia, and, if left unchecked for a number of years, can develop into cancer of the uterus.

Transdermal progesterone has been shown to reverse the effects of estrogen stimulation of the uterine lining, but does require measurement of levels or sampling of the uterine lining. I typically measure the level of progesterone 12 hours after application of the cream or ingestion of the pill.

These levels are not all that important in the context of estrogen dominance, as we are not giving estrogen to the patient and therefore do not need to worry about inducing endometrial hyperplasia. We will discuss progesterone levels in detail in a later chapter.

It is important to remember that estrogen dominance is simply the balance of these hormones in relationship to each other. It does not describe the overall level of estrogen in the body. It is possible to have low, normal or high levels of estrogen in the setting of estrogen dominance.

This is often confusing to patients who interpret estrogen dominance as meaning high overall levels of estrogen, which is why it's important to remember that hormones can be in or out of balance with each other – in addition to their absolute levels in an individual.

DIET AND ESTROGEN DOMINANCE

Other interventions can be used to combat and avoid estrogen dominance. One is our diet, which is often compromised. As a society, we have allowed industrial concerns free rein to make changes to our foods. Too often, these changes have involved the addition of chemicals and preservatives in order to prolong shelf life and appearance. Many of these chemicals have not been adequately tested for their effects on our hormone systems.

Meanwhile, the whole area of xenoestrogen is rapidly developing and may be more important than we realize at this time.

My recommendation for most people is to eat natural foods, grown within 100 miles of your home address, and to minimize the preservatives you ingest. Certified organic foods usually fit the bill and are worth the extra expense. Next best would be to add fruits and vegetables in their natural state, with attention to proper preparation of them to minimize herbicide and pesticide exposure. Below is a vegetable and fruit wash that has been proven very effective in doing so.

Detox Bath Recipe

1 cup pickling salt

½ cup baking soda

2 good shots of peroxide

Diet can also be used to select foods with natural abilities to reduce estrogen dominance. Indole-3-carbinol (I3C) and di-indoyl-methane (DIMM) are compounds derived from the brassica group of vegetables, which includes broccoli, cabbage and cauliflower. These vegetables seem to have inherent cancer fighting properties, due to their effects on estrogen metabolism or breakdown. If you are not crazy about these vegetables, the compounds themselves are available in supplement form.

Estrogen, when produced or ingested, needs to be removed from the body or it will accumulate to toxic levels. Estrogen metabolism involves attaching chemical side-chains to estrogen in the liver. These modifications allow the body to excrete the hormones in the stool and urine. Some metabolites are safe, and some are more dangerous than the hormone itself. I believe the fact that many families seem to be prone to certain cancers relates to their hormone metabolism. These families will have an inherited problem in hormone metabolism that will cause them to produce more of the harmful hormone metabolites.

DIMM and 13C have powerful effects on hormone metabolism. We will discuss them at length in the next chapter, but here's a brief summary: DIMM is easily absorbed in supplement form and shifts estrogen metabolism down the cancer-protective 2-hydroxy pathway.

Xenoestrogens in the form of chlorinated pesticides and organopesticides reduce 2-hydroxy estrogen metabolism and increase 16 hydroxy estrogen metabolic products, which are genotoxic to our DNA and increase cancer formation. DIMM can be used in supplement form to increase 2-hydroxylation of estrogen and reduce cancer risk.

There is much more to the story of hormones and cancer risk than meets the eye. Our approach to date has been far too simplistic. It is time to wake up and use all available approaches to reduce the incidence of this terrible affliction. BHRT is one of the modalities I believe we can use while improving quality of life. A doctor knowledgeable in this area can measure hormone metabolism and prescribe supplementation to increase the formation of healthy metabolites and reduce formation of the harmful ones.

Our livers are working overtime to eliminate the toxins we absorb. The body also can excrete toxins through sweat and reduce the toxic load on the liver. Infrared saunas directly increase sweating and toxin excretion, and are an excellent way to improve health. Dr. Sherry Rogers' book *Detoxify or Die* is an excellent resource for more information on how to approach detoxification.

REAL WOMEN, REAL STORIES

L.G.

After hearing my numerous concerns, Dr. Brown asked, "Is there anything else?"

"Well, I don't sleep very well." was my reply. I would typically get between four or five hours of sleep a night before I would awaken, usually around 3 a.m. I had thought it was a result of years of broken sleep from raising our three children. Despite applying all the good sleep hygiene suggestions that I had learned about, I still couldn't get a decent night's sleep. I was frustrated and I blamed myself.

"I think I can help" Dr. Brown stated quietly. Those words changed my life.

I was prescribed Prometrium, a bioidentical hormone, and within two weeks I started sleeping 7 to 7½ hours continuously. I was amazed that it was that easy. It was simply delicious to sleep like that again.

The change that it made in my life was profound. I was more patient and tolerant with my kids, who were now teenagers. I had more energy to exercise and I could even stay awake past 10 p.m. to enjoy the other benefits of having my hormones balanced. That one result has snowballed into many very good changes in my life.

Important Points

1. Estrogen production is stable from age 25 to menopause.

2. Progesterone production falls 50% from age 20 to 40, and continues to decline till menopause.

3. The increase in estrogen relative to progesterone creates estrogen dominance in the late 30s and 40s.

4. Estrogen dominance is increased with obesity and exposure to phthalates in plastics.

5. Estrogen dominance can present as:

    • Anxiety and panic attacks

    • Depression and irritability

    • Insomnia

    • Pain as a result of joint and body inflammation

    • Bloating

    • Heavy menstrual bleeding

    • Carbohydrate cravings

    • Tender, fibrocystic breasts

    • Migraine headaches

6. The dictum "No uterus – no progesterone" is false and misleading. A woman has many tissues dependent on progesterone in addition to the uterus.

7. The treatments of estrogen dominance are diet, exercise and progesterone

8. Progesterone can be prescribed as a pill or cream.

9. Proper diet selection and preparation, toxin avoidance, and infrared saunas can be used to decrease the exposure to environmental xenoestrogens that worsen estrogen dominance.

CHAPTER 7

ESTROGENS: THE GOOD, BAD AND THE UGLY

After our discussion on estrogen dominance, you may be wondering why we even look at estrogen in HRT. Certainly, before menopause, there is very little need for estrogen. With the dramatic fall in estrogen as a result of the menopausal transition, estrogen therapy is commonly required for SYMPTOMATIC women. At this point in time there is no scientific evidence that estrogen therapy prolongs life. Many BHRT practitioners feel that BHRT will result in life extension, but we are really only certain that it improves quality of life at this time. BHRT uses a combination of estriol(protective) and estradiol(effective) to treat symptoms in symptomatic, post-menopausal women. This choice is due to some of the remarkable attributes of estriol that warrant a re-examination of its role in hormone replacement therapy. We will discuss these special qualities of estriol in this chapter.

If you ask a conventional gynecologist about estrogen replacement therapy, he/she will probably tell you that there is no debate. Estradiol, or a modified estradiol, will be suggested as the estrogen drug of choice. In fact, you'll probably be told that estradiol is a bioidentical hormone and the only one needed for HRT. I disagree and hope to convince you of this as well, by the end of this chapter.

While it is true that estradiol is a bioidentical hormone, that is not the most important part of the story. In fact, once most people learn the real facts about the little-known estrogen called estriol, their outlook is forever changed.

As we've mentioned in other chapters, up to menopause, almost all women have adequate levels of estrogen. However, at the time of menopause, a woman's estrogen production falls drastically. During this transition, testosterone production is stable and progesterone production only falls to a small extent.

And in many cases, estrogen-deprivation symptoms suddenly rise to the forefront and produce a dramatic decline in the quality of life.

Common estrogen-deficiency symptoms include:

Hot Flashes	Night Sweats
Memory Problems	Painful Intercourse
Bladder Infections	Depression
Decreased Energy	

Table 7-1: Estrogen deficiency

Of course, the occurrences of these symptoms, like many others, will depend on a number of factors that can be independent of the menopause transition.

For example, in most cases, thin women with low amounts of body fat will suffer the symptoms of estrogen deprivation more severely. This is usually because a lower amount of body fat reduces the body's capacity to convert adrenal androgens such as androstenedione into estrogen. Conversely, many overweight women will have no symptoms of estrogen deficiency as they move into menopause.

It's important to remember, however, that every woman is an individual. That's why I – along with a growing number of respected colleagues – believe the medical profession needs to discard the one-size-fits-all approach to hormone-replacement therapy. When we stop practicing what amounts to cookie-cutter medicine, and take the time to develop an individualized approach to each woman's unique metabolism, she usually sees almost dramatic results, with the ultimate effect of a better quality of life.

LET'S TALK ABOUT ESTROGEN AND RECEPTORS

The body produces three types of estrogen, and each is strongest at different times in a woman's life.

Estradiol (E2) is produced primarily by the ovaries, and is strongest during the premenopausal period, when a woman is in her child-bearing years. It is the estrogen of youth and is responsible for much of what makes a woman feel like a woman. The loss of estradiol production at menopause is responsible for most of the estrogen-deprivation symptoms we associate with menopause.

Estriol (E3) is produced by the placenta and is the dominant form of estrogen during pregnancy.

The third form is estrone (E1), which becomes dominant after menopause, and is made primarily through the conversion of androstenedione to estrone in fat cells.

There are two main estrogen-receptor types in the human body – alpha and beta. Each has different effects when stimulated by estrogen. The estrogen-alpha receptor (ER-A) increases cell growth, including those of breast cells. The estrogen-beta receptor (ER-B) inhibits breast-cell growth because of its effect on cell replication. These two receptors are distributed in different parts of the body to produce the desired effects on those tissues.

The three estrogens have different binding affinities to each of the two receptors – and therefore the results or effects of hormone therapy are dictated by the way a particular estrogen interacts with these two seperate estrogen receptors. Sadly, the conventional medical community has largely overlooked this fact, mostly because of the patent law discussed in Chapter 4. The pharmaceutical industry has always focused on estradiol for its products. I can't stress enough that this issue is at the center of the whole debate on BHRT.

PHARMACEUTICAL PRODUCTS AND ESTRADIOL

All pharmaceutical products related to this field are estradiol-focused, and all have suffered by being associated with increased risks of breast cancer. I know there will be skeptical physicians reading this, especially as what I'm saying is contrary to the teaching of the day. That is why I've taken the time and trouble to provide references from recent scientific literature – to give these skeptics scientific support for my position.

Estradiol, the primary estrogen produced by premenopausal women, is a very powerful hormone that has an equal stimulation effect on both ER-A and ER-B receptors. Remember, the A receptor causes tissue growth and the B receptor prevents tissue growth. Cancer is a manifestation of too much growth. With estrogen, we are primarily talking about overgrowth leading to cancer of the breast.

Estradiol's effect on receptor stimulation is a 1:1 ratio when we look at A and B estrogen receptor stimulation, and that's the main reason it's so powerful for symptom relief. In contrast, estriol selectively binds ER-B in a 3:1 ratio[1], resulting in much less breast cell growth. This gives estriol a significant breast protection effect. In fact, a study has shown that estriol, when given with estradiol, has a unique ability to protect breast tissue from excess estradiol-mediated stimulation[2].

When it acts alone, estriol is a weak estrogen, but when given with estradiol, it becomes an anti-estrogen. This is because when estriol binds to the receptor in a tissue responsive to estrogen, it stimulates the receptor target very weakly. Estriol's presence and receptor binding prevents the two stronger estrogens from binding to the receptor.[3] This is called the "Estriol Hypothesis" which to date has not received much attention in the conventional hormone literature. Can patent considerations be at the heart of this apparent disregard for what appears to be a safer approach to estrogen replacement therapy? This is called competitive antagonism and is used extensively in BHRT. Estriol reduces activated receptors from binding to estrogen-response elements on the DNA, and this limits the gene transcription. Less gene transcription means less protein production and a milder effect of the hormone overall. Estrone has not been used in BHRT in recent years mainly because it[3] selectively activates ER-A in a 5:1 ratio[4].

Estriol production increases 1,000 times and progesterone production increases 15 times in pregnancy. The increase in progesterone helps to allow implantation and growth of the developing embryo. Increased estriol may have effects on placental metabolism. The net effect of these hormone changes is protection against breast cancer development.

After giving birth, new mothers continue to produce higher levels of estriol than women who have never been pregnant[5]. This significant and long-term exposure to estriol and progesterone provides a significant reduction in the long-term risk of breast cancer[6].

In fact, probably one of the most important studies of the benefits of estriol and progesterone was presented at the September 2002 meeting of the U.S. Department of Defense Breast Cancer Research Meeting.

Dr. P. Sliiteri, an investigator on the effects of hormones in pregnancy on breast cancer, and his colleagues performed a 40-year longitudinal study on 15,000 women in the Kaiser Foundation Health Plan. Blood was taken from pregnant women, stored for up to 20 years, and then analyzed for hormone levels using modern methods. These hormone levels were then compared with the California Cancer Registry and breast cancer in particular.

Only estriol, out of all the sex hormones measured in these pregnant women, was linked with development of breast cancer in later life. The women with high estriol production had a 58% reduced risk of breast cancer as compared with those who produced low levels of estriol in pregnancy[7]. I've found at least 10 other studies confirming that highestriol levels in pregnancy confer a reduced risk of breast cancer in later life.

This raises the question: If the benefits of E3 are so strongly supported, why is there opposition to its use in HRT?

The answer, unfortunately, lies in the patent issue. The problem is, as of the writing of this book, no one has discovered a substitute for E3 that can be patented. No patent means no profit – and without the profit potential, there's no research into the benefits. After all, what's the point of sponsoring research into a compound that can't be put on the market?

But as the results of just the studies I've illustrated above show, there are some compelling reasons to use estriol as part of a hormone-replacement therapy program to reduce the incidence of breast cancer.

In Western Europe, estriol has been used for many years for this purpose[8]. In fact, it is produced by a major pharmaceutical company, Organon, as a prescription cream in Europe called Ovestin. Unfortunately, in North America, the pharmaceutical companies have taken a different approach and have tried to have estriol banned as an estrogenic agent for HRT.

Estriol has a number of other functions, [9] which include:

Rejuvenates the vaginal lining	Decreases LDL, one of the bad cholesterol components
Controls symptoms of menopause	Restores proper vaginal PH, reducing the number of urinary-tract infections
Increases HDL, the beneficial form of cholesterol	Reduces appearance of wrinkles and fine lines, makes skin look younger, no more dull, brittle hair

Table 7-2: Estriol's benefits

As we can see, estriol has a number of beneficial effects and no known negative properties. Its safety and efficacy have been extensively studied as far back as 30 years ago, with no caution other than slight thickening of the uterine lining, which requires monitoring[10,11].

In a 1980 review, Wolf Utian, founder of the North American Menopause Society, reported estriol to have similar benefits to other estrogens with a potential for decreased risk of breast cancer development.[12]

Estriol's effects on the estrogen receptor are most interesting. Estriol (E3) plays an important role in the normal balance of estrogens in the body. Both estradiol (E2) and estrone (E1) are much stronger estrogens than estriol, and strongly bind to the alpha estrogen receptor, resulting in a proliferation inducing effect. E3 can act as both an estrogen and anti-estrogen by competitively inhibiting E2 and E3 estrogen receptor binding[13].

The way that E1 and E2 strongly bind and stimulate the alpha estrogen receptor creates breast cell growth. E3 on the other hand, selectively binds the beta estrogen receptor in a 3:1 ratio and possesses significant potential for breast cancer protection. Since estriol can bind the alpha receptor but only produces a weak effect, the net result is that estriol reduces the stronger actions of estradiol and estrone on the estrogen receptor when they are used together. Numerous studies show a reduced risk of breast cancer with E3 use. These studies are well detailed in an extensive review on E3 by Jim Paoletti this year[13].

Tamoxifen is an estrogenic substance that works by the same mechanism as E3, and is promoted as an anti-estrogen. Tamoxifen, unfortunately, has some potentially serious long-term side effects that limit its use. Estriol has none of these safety concerns making it easy to understand why it is preferred in Europe for protection in breast cancer survivors.

The estrogen receptor is a rather complex structure that deserves some attention[1,4,13]. Two estrogen molecules bound to two estrogen receptors to form a dimer receptor complex (dimer is a scientific term for pair) that then acts on DNA within a cell nucleus. This dimeric receptor complex binds to specific spots on certain hormone response genes and initiates a response. The gene response is to start producing a protein that then goes on to have effects on cell metabolism.

Therefore, two estrogen molecules are required to form the dimer receptor complex and initiate protein translation. The strength of an estrogen depends on how tightly it binds to the receptor. The stronger the binding, the longer the estrogen molecule remains bound to the receptor complex and the more protein translation occurs and the stronger the effect of that hormone. Once one of the estrogen molecules separates from the receptor complex, the gene translation and message stops.

Since E3 weakly attaches to the alpha receptor, it is able to soften the message sent by E2. The more E3 that's present, the weaker the stimulation effect of E1 and E2. The competitive effect of E3 on E2 is quite a bit more complicated than this simple explanation, and a detailed account is outlined in the paper by Melamed[3].

This effect forms the basis of the rationale to use a product called Biest in BHRT. Biest is a combination of E2 and E3 with variable proportions of the two estrogens in question. I prefer an 80:20 Biest, with

80% E3 and 20% E2, as the patient is more likely to experience all the benefits of E3 with this ratio.

In the past, a compound called Triest was used for BHRT. Triest is a combination of E1, E2 and E3. Estrone (E1) is a weak estrogen that has a particular affinity with the alpha estrogen receptor. This affinity has been shown to predispose E1 to increasing the risk of uterine cancer.

Since E1 has no beneficial properties and some downside risk, I can't support its use in BHRT. I recommend that patients on Triest switch to the safer and equally effective Biest preparation.

The above discussion may seem complicated to the average reader but it only really scratches the surface of the complexities of estrogen action.

The predominant estrogen in non-pregnant women is E1. In pregnant women E3 is the dominant estrogen. The concentrations of these estrogens relative to E2 in the pregnant and non-pregnant state determine the overall effect of estrogen in those women.

Estradiol and estrone are able to convert back and forth in manners that we do not completely understand. Estriol is unique, in that once it is formed it can't be converted back to estradiol or estrone. This may in part confer estriol its beneficial effects. As this knowledge develops, there are sure to be new chapters written on the effects of the different estrogens in women.

Suffice it to say that at this time estriol appears to be an important part of BHRT strategy to reduce the risk of breast cancer. To say this whole area has been overlooked is an understatement. One of the observations of the WHI study was that there was a decreased incidence of breast cancer in the Premarin-only treatment arm. This observation flies in the face of generally held beliefs of estrogen and breast cancer. The prevailing belief is that estrogen therapy increases the risk of breast cancer. How can we resolve this apparent contradiction? I have asked this question of a number of reproductive endocrinologists and have never received an answer to explain the reduced breast cancer incidence in the Premarin only arm. All of the analysis of the WHI has failed to address this issue. Premarin is an unique estrogen compound and one of the constituents is 17-alpha-dihydroequilin(17ADEQ). 17ADEQ makes up 15% of Premarin and has no estrogenic and some apparent anti-estrogenic activity. Is it possible that the reduction in risk of breast cancer seen with Premarin alone in the WHI is a result of this little known horse estrogen? Is it possible that estriol can have a similar effect as 17ADEQ when used as a human identical hormone in a BHRT program? At this time we have more questions than answers, but there seems to be great merit in these questions. Why is no one else asking the questions??

Part of the difficulty is that the picture becomes even muddier when we look at estrogen metabolism. The body has to find a way to inactivate and excrete all hormone compounds used in metabolism. The liver is the site of hormone metabolism and eventual excretion of the deactivated hormones.

First a hormone goes through Phase 1 detoxification, where a molecule is attached to the hormone to make it more water-soluble. Phase 2 of detoxification involves attaching another molecule to the altered hormone to allow its excretion into and out of the digestive tract. Once excreted into the stool through the bile, hormones exit the body in stool.

Phase 1 detoxification results in a number of different molecules for each of the different estrogens. The balance of the different metabolites can increase or decrease the risk of cancer formation. This means we should have at least a basic understanding of the issues regarding estrogen metabolism.

Phase 1 detoxification of estrogens results in three main pathways.

1. 2-hydroxylation

2. 4-hydroxylation

3. 16-hydroxylation

Phase 1 metabolites are hormones in their own right and have powerful effects in the body. In fact, some Phase 1 products are stronger than the original hormone they came from. The 2-hydroxylation pathway, results in compounds that protect against cancer formation. Therefore, we would like to ensure that the body uses this detoxification pathway as much as possible. The 4- and 16-hydroxylation products are cancer-promoting pathways and are best to be minimized.

It is possible to measure the relative proportions of these pathways in the urine and determine whether an individual's Phase 1 pathways are putting her at risk of cancer. These products are measured in a urine test called a 2/16 ratio. The higher the 2/16 ratio, the smaller the risk of cancer. We always like to see the ratio higher than 1.0.

I like to measure the ratio once a particular dose of BHRT has been found to improve a patient's symptoms. Once we have someone feeling better, it's good to know that she is not at increased risk of cancer based on her hormone metabolism.

If we find a low 2/16 ratio, DIMM (di-indoylmethane) and I3C (indole-3-carbinol) can be prescribed to increase the 2/16 ratio. Indole-3-carbinol is a precursor indole of the brassica family of vegetables (cabbage, broccoli and cauliflower), and was used in the past for this effect.

Unfortunately, I3C is erratically absorbed and has an inconsistent effect. DIMM appears to be better absorbed and produces a more consistent improvement in the 2/16 ratio.

As we can see, there is much to consider when it comes to estrogen therapy.

Unfortunately conventional gynecology has approached the area in a very simplistic fashion.

I believe this is in large part due to the strong influence of the pharmaceutical industry on medical research and treatment in North America. Europe has a much more balanced approach to the area, and we have much to learn from that. I trust that in the fullness of time, BHRT will lead us to a more open-minded outlook on estrogen-replacement therapy, an approach that puts patient safety ahead of commercial interests.

Important Points

1. Estrogen production falls dramatically at the menopausal transition and can produce many unpleasant symptoms.

2. Thin women suffer the symptoms of estrogen-deprivation to a greater extent than overweight women.

3. There are three estrogens:

    - Estrone (E1): weak estrogen with cancer-promoting properties

    - Estradiol (E2): strong estrogen that promotes cell growth, especially in the breast

    - Estriol (E3): weak estrogen with breast cancer-fighting properties

4. There are two estrogen receptors:

    - Alpha: stimulation induces cell proliferation

    - Beta: stimulation is considered anti-proliferative

5. Estrogen receptors are not randomly distributed. Different tissues have different relative concentrations of the two receptors. The balance of the receptors in a tissue determines estrogen effects on that tissue.

6. Each estrogen has a different affinity for each of the estrogen receptors.

7. Estriol has a stronger affinity for the beta receptor and can also act as a mild anti-estrogen due to its competition with estradiol.

8. Estriol reduces the risk of breast cancer.

9. BHRT uses estriol along with estradiol as its estrogen-treatment agent. This is expected to reduce the chances of breast cancer with estrogen-replacement in BHRT.

10. Estrogen metabolism creates different compounds that can increase or decrease the risk of breast cancer.

11. The 2/16 ration for estrogen metabolism can be measured in women. BHRT increases the 2/16 ratio and decreases the risk of breast cancer.

1 Zhu, BT et al. Endocrinology 2006; 147 (9) 4132-50 / 2 Lemon, BM et al. Acta Endocrinol Suppl 1980; 233: 17-27
3 Melamed, M et al. Mol Endocrinol 1997; 11(12) 1868-78 / 4 Rich, R L et al. Proc Natl Acad Sci USA 2002; 99 (13)
8562-7 / 5 Speroff, L Contemp Obstet Gynec 1977; 9: 69-72 / 6 Innes, KE et al. Int J Cancer 2004 112(2) 306-11
7 Sliiteri, P K et al. / 8 Head, K Altern Med Review 1998; 3: 101-13 / 9 Holtorf, K Post Grad Med 2009; 121: 1-13
10 Takahashi, K et al. Hum Reprod 2000; 15 (5): 1028-36 / 11 Manonai, J et al. J med Assoc Thai 200; 84 (4): 539-44
12 Utian, WH Acta Endocrinol Suppl (Copenh) 1980; 233: 51-5 / 13 Paoletti, J   Int J Pharm Comp 2009; 13 (4) 270-5
14 Speroff, L et al. Clinical End.

CHAPTER 8

PROGESTERONE: NATURE'S BALANCING AGENT

A SHORT AND FASCINATING LOOK AT THE HISTORY OF MEDICINE

In her book *Chinese Civilization: A Sourcebook*, Patricia Buckley Ebrey says, "The concepts of Yin and Yang and the Five Agents provided the intellectual framework of much of Chinese scientific thinking especially in fields like biology and medicine. The organs of the body were seen to be interrelated in the same sorts of ways as other natural phenomena, and best understood by looking for correlations and correspondences.

"Illness was seen as a disturbance in the balance of Yin and Yang or the Five Agents caused by emotions, heat or cold, or other influences. Therapy thus depended on accurate diagnosis of the source of the imbalance ... "

From a historical perspective, I find it fascinating that the earliest surviving medical texts are fragments of manuscript from early Han tombs. Besides general theory, these texts cover the gamut of medical knowledge and practice of the day – everything from drugs to gymnastics, minor surgery to magic spells.

The text – which was to become the main source of medical theory – apparently dates from the Han, during the Third Millennium, and written by the mythical "Yellow Emperor." He said, "The principle of Yin and Yang is the foundation of the entire universe. It underlies everything in creation. It brings about the development of parenthood; it is the root and source of life and death …

"In order to treat and cure diseases one must search for their origins … If Yang is overly powerful, then Yin may be too weak. If Yin is particularly strong, then Yang is apt to be defective. Thus Yin and Yang alternate. Their ebbs and surges vary, and so does the character of the diseases … "

FINDING BALANCE IN THE MODERN WORLD

This need for balance is a recurring theme in the study of nature and the way all systems are structured. If you look at anthropology, biology, chemistry, ecology, environmental science, genetics or any other branch of study, there always has to be balance to keep a system running smoothly and at optimum levels. And we've certainly found this to be true with our own bodies, our health and the aging process. For hormones, there is no better example of this than the balance of estrogen and progesterone.

In the previous chapter, you read that estrogen in its various forms is primarily a force of proliferation and growth. When left uncontrolled – which causes a systemic imbalance – this force creates the potential for cancer, which is uncontrolled growth.

Why would nature allow such a situation to occur? The answer lies in the very mechanism – the method – of reproduction. Almost all hormones feed back on their receptors in a negative fashion. In other words, as the concentration of a hormone increases, it reduces the ability of its receptor to react to it over time, and less of that hormone receptor is expressed in the cell. This is an example of the balance inherent in natural systems.

Only estrogen and its receptor interaction fail to follow this plan. Why would there be an exception? Early in its development, a female fetus carries numerous follicles, or potential eggs, in its ovaries. A large proportion of those follicles are lost before birth. More of the potential eggs are lost before the female starts to menstruate. And then, once her periods start, each month a large number of the remaining ovarian follicles start to develop – each one hoping to become "the" egg.

Of course, it wouldn't be a good thing for women to have hundreds of fertilized eggs, so nature created a way to select only the strongest and healthiest of these competing ovarian follicles – a kind of beauty pageant, if you will. The system allows estrogen to increase the number and sensitivity of its own receptors.

This means the developing eggs "compete" with one another to produce more estrogen and therefore more receptors. And as the competition continues, the weaker of the developing follicles are shut down, one after another, until only one remains. And as the "winner," it's released in ovulation, and with the intention of being fertilized.

In scientific terminology, this is called the two-cell hypothesis of reproduction, and if you're interested, it's been well-outlined in many reproductive endocrinology medical texts. For our purposes, the details of the competition are of no real interest, but the concept of a "positive-feed forward loop" of estrogen is – because it explains why estrogen is the only hormone able to increase the number and sensitivity of its own receptors and why, without this ability, reproduction would not be possible.

Logic would dictate that if a system was developed that could not naturally control itself, then another system – an opposing force, if you will – must be designed to control the first system. That's where progesterone comes in. Progesterone is the opposing force to estrogen, and we see it in the interplay between the two hormones every month.

Through the first half of the cycle, estrogen production steadily increases the growth of the uterine lining in anticipation of a fertilized egg implantation, fulfilling estrogen's function of causing proliferation.

PROGESTERONE'S ROLE BEFORE MENOPAUSE

Once ovulation occurs, the corpus luteum begins to steadily increase the production of progesterone to counteract the effects of estrogen stimulation on the uterine lining. Progesterone also prepares the uterus for the implantation of the egg, helps to support and maintain the pregnancy, and, equally important, prevents further ovulation during the rest of the pregnancy.

Even with high estrogen levels, progesterone is able to reverse the proliferation effects of estrogen. If, after 14 days, there is no fertilized egg, the woman has a period, which brings the uterine lining back to normal, and stops the uncontrolled growth.

The medical field has known for many years that unopposed production or use of estrogen will always lead to uterine cancer. Unfortunately, gynecology also had a kind of tunnel vision when it came to

women and estrogen. We have also known for many years that progesterone can deplete the number of estrogen receptors in a given tissue by
accelerating the destruction of estrogen receptors. Plus, progesterone
reduces the creation of new estrogen receptors by blocking estrogen's
actions on genes responsible for production of estrogen receptors[1].
Decreased estrogen receptors means reduced sensitivity of that tissue's
cells to estrogen. Progesterone is the Yin to estrogen's Yang!

PROGESTERONE AFTER CHILD-BEARING YEARS

As mentioned before, Wyeth was the first company to produce
estrogen for women, in the form of Premarin. It was a huge breakthrough and benefited millions of women over the years. Unfortunately, after years of Premarin being used alone as unopposed estrogen,
we discovered that it dramatically increased the risk of uterine cancer.

We now understand estrogen's role in cell proliferation. As an
estrogen-sensitive tissue, the uterus needs a monthly exposure to
adequate levels of progesterone to prevent ongoing cell growth and
cancer development. Once this was determined, a progesterone-like
compound, or progestin, was developed. This compound was called
Provera, and was patented for use with Premarin. At that time, natural
progesterone could not be administered in a pill form because stomach
acid destroyed the progesterone before it could be absorbed in the
small intestine.

Around the time of the Women's Health Initiative debacle, a
French company had developed a way to put natural progesterone into
microsomes. These microsomes were resistant to stomach acid and
allowed the use of progesterone as a pill. This drug is called Prome-

trium, and it and a compounded, micronized progesterone are used extensively in BHRT.

Other research found that progesterone could be absorbed through the skin in a transdermal preparation.

The problem for the WHI was that the sponsoring company, Wyeth, did not own the patent on Prometrium, and a patent could not be granted to trans-dermal progesterone. So investigators went with their own formulation, medroxyprogesterone acetate or PMA, and the rest is history. We can only wonder what the WHI would have shown if Prometrium had been chosen as the progestational agent. Perhaps HRT would be seen in a favorable light these days, rather than an unsafe approach to feeling better.

We discussed that progesterone production declines from age 25 to 50. We have also seen that estrogen production is well maintained over these years, setting up the estrogen dominance problem discussed in Chapter 6. Also, the natural tendency for weight gain is compounded by environmental xenoestrogens exposure. All of these factors set up a progesterone-deficiency problem of enormous proportions.

What does progesterone deficiency look like?
- PMS
- Insomnia
- Painful, lumpy breasts
- Unexplained weight gain
- Cyclic headaches
- Anxiety
- Infertility

You probably notice that this list looks a lot like the symptoms of estrogen dominance. In fact, the two are almost indistinguishable on the basis of symptoms. The only way to determine your level of estrogen is to have a blood, saliva or urine test. A test to determine your progesterone level can be done at the same time. At this point, your doctor will ask you questions about your symptoms in order to determine your estrogen/progesterone balance.

In the luteal phase of the menstrual cycle, a woman makes approximately 30 mg of progesterone per day. Doses around this level are common in transdermal therapy. We know that progesterone is safe at doses much higher than this from the study of progesterone in pregnancy. In the third trimester, progesterone production can reach 400 mg per day. Even at these doses, we see no adverse effects in the woman or fetus.

WHEN "NATURAL" PROGESTERONE ISN'T

Unfortunately the same cannot be said for progestins like Provera or medroxyprogesterone acetate. There was an increased risk of minor birth defects in children of women who prescribed Provera in early pregnancy to reduce the risk of miscarriage. And, studies done with beagle puppies showed an increased risk of breast nodules, some of which were malignant with the use of Provera on a continual basis.

So why do we persist with progestins now that natural progesterone is available? Sadly, I think we all know that answer by now! I want to remind you that "natural" progesterone is still synthetic. Remember that while it is, in fact, human-identical, it is certainly NOT natural! Progesterone is synthesized from diogensin, a compound derived from the Mexican yam or soybeans. Through a series of chemical reactions, diogensin is converted into estradiol, estriol, testosterone and progesterone.

While not natural, all of these steroid hormones used in BHRT are human-identical and work as nature intended them in the body. It is the practitioner's job to establish the proper balance in a patient. It is the proper balance and levels of these human-identical hormones that provides the safety in this form of HRT.

Many examples in medical literature today show how imbalances of these hormones lead to disease and cancer. While there is greater inherent safety of these hormones compared with their pharmaceutical look-alikes, proper levels and balances must be obtained to ensure safety.

Some companies try to sell diogensin as "wild yam extract." They claim the body can convert the diogensin into the hormones as needed. *But these are false claims and the necessary conversions will not take place in the body.* I do not recommend the use of "wild yam" cream in light of the ready availability of progesterone cream and pills.

WHAT MATTERS:

Progesterone: A hormone produced in the ovaries, the placenta (during pregnancy), and the adrenal glands and stored in fat tissue. Progesterone travels through the blood to tissues that hold its receptors, and works to control and turn off estrogen, and other "work" in the body.

Progestin: A synthetic form of progesterone whose structure has been chemically altered.

Corpus luteum: The corpus luteum, which means "yellow body" in Latin, is what is left of the follicle after a woman ovulates.

Ovulation: Ovulation occurs when a mature egg is released from the ovary, pushed down the fallopian tube and is available to be fertilized.

Annovulatory cycle: A menstrual cycle in which ovulation fails to occur. This means that you do bleed but do not release an egg or ovulate.

Provera: A progestin that has progesterone-like effects on the uterus, but has a chemical structure different from progesterone. Manufactured in a laboratory and derived either from progesterone (usually equine) or from testosterone. The testosterone-derived progestins have more androgenic properties.

Premarin: The commercial name for a compound drug consisting primarily of conjugated estrogens. Isolated from mare's urine (PREgnant MARe 's urINe), it is manufactured by Wyeth Pharmaceuticals (part of Pfizer since January 2009).

REAL WOMEN, REAL STORIES

J.C.

One of my passions is planting and tending to my garden. A long time ago a friend said to me that the best time to plant a tree was 20 years ago and the next best time is now.

The philosophy of making each day an important step in the rest of your life is one that I have taken to heart. Without question, the same applies to Dr. Brown and how his clinic and expertise has improved the quality of my life. I am 49 years old and have been seeing Dr. Brown for seven short months.

I am thankful for the first day that I planted the seed on my journey to wellness as I cannot imagine the alternative. A miracle, I don't think so, but it sure feels like one! Now I need to take you back in time...

I am not sure when I started feeling poorly, but it was a long time ago. It began with profoundly heavy periods that seemed to worsen with each passing month.

I was sent for several ultrasounds due to what my family doctor referred to as controlled hemorrhaging. It reached a point where I no longer had monthly cycles, just one continuous, painful period. This persisted for several years until I felt I had no other option than to undergo a total hysterectomy. Soon thereafter, the discomfort of my period was replaced by severe headaches, hot flashes and periodic night sweats.

Over a period of five years, the night sweats progressed to a level that did not allow for any suitable sleeping pattern. I consulted with my family doctor several times but only left the office with recommendations of over-the-counter remedies. I faithfully tried them all only to confirm that these did not work for me.

It is not over-exaggerating to say I was exhausted 24 hours a day … it was so difficult to get out of bed in the morning and once I did, I couldn't allow myself to stop during the day as I was certain that I could not get up again.

In retrospect, I was robotic because it was the only way I could function. My family told me I didn't smile and I never understood them at the time.

This was not how I viewed myself, but admittedly, I had lost myself and did not realize it. I am a professional woman with a demanding career, I am a mother who loves and cares for her sons, aged 15 and 23, I am a woman who loves her husband, what more could anyone want of me? I was certain of one thing though… I didn't know what it felt like to be well and it seemed I spent my waking hours on autopilot.

I am a big believer that things happen for a reason. Having said this, I didn't seek out Dr. Brown for his expertise in BHRT. A good friend of mine told me of a Dr. Brown in Sherwood Park that she had heard of through friends. I made a phone call which ultimately ended up in my enrollment in a Spring Health Symposium at True Balance.

This was not a researched decision on my part. I had not heard of BHRT until the day of the symposium. I sat through the presentations until my scheduled appointment with Dr. Brown at 3:30 p.m. It was only at this point that I realized each session presented was relevant to my purpose in being here. After my appointment with Dr. Brown, I was consumed with the need to leave his office immediately.

I was overwhelmed with the realization that everything I had been feeling was real and apparently treatable.

Here was this guy, telling me I would be shocked from the results after two months of treatment. I remember telling Dr. Brown that "pleasantly pleased" would be sufficient. I also realized that the pain I felt on the inside was outward facing.

Although I held a healthy skepticism of what might come to be, I remember feeling that this interaction with Dr. Brown was vastly different from any I had experienced before.

For the first time, I felt diagnosed and understood. The completeness of the blood work ordered by Dr. Brown addressed issues and prescribed remedies that should have been diagnosed by my family physician who I was faithful in seeing several times throughout the years.

As Dr. Brown avowed during my first appointment, I was truly shocked by the results. Within two weeks I was feeling better. Within a month, others around me noticed the difference and began to comment. Within three months I had found me again. Within three months! I had literally spent years trying to achieve this state, feeling like it was an unachievable goal. I remember telling Dr. Brown on my first follow-up appointment, "I just feel like me."

Feeling like me again is a great thing! What I feel on the inside shows on the outside! I have an abundance of energy, plenty of smiles, laughter, and a zest for the journey I take each and every day.

What was remarkable was how many people noticed a difference. Family members, work associates, my hairdresser, my esthetician, my massage therapist, my family doctor and friend after friend commented on my beautiful skin, my bright eyes, my energy, my smile, and in general how great I was looking.

I know looking great starts on the inside and works its way to the surface but this transformation happened in such a short period of time. Remarkable!

For me, the most profound changes were in how I felt and how I continue to feel. I am no longer plagued by headaches. My brain is clearer in that I can again make conscious decisions in what I do or choose not to do, whether it is in my professional life or my home life. My energy level is where I expect it to be and I can easily manage my full days. I sleep at night ... hooray! My sex drive is back, much to my delight, and I have not had one hot flash or night sweat since two weeks after I began my program.

The transformation from my inside to my outside was so profound that I cannot even count the friends, friends of friends, family members and acquaintances who have visited Dr. Brown since I started. My husband just began his program this past month as this is one journey we definitely want to share.

Like gardening, this journey to wellness has been incredibly rewarding ... you plant a seed, you nurture it with what it needs to thrive, and you watch it flourish. Life doesn't get better than this!

Important Facts

1. The concept of "balance" has strong historical roots and has been recognized over the millennia.

2. Estrogen is the only hormone that can increase the concentration of its own receptors.

3. Progesterone is able to decrease estrogen receptors and hasten the destruction of estrogen in the cell.

4. Provera is NOT progesterone.

5. From age 20 to 50, woman have a significant reduction in progesterone production. This creates estrogen dominance.

6. Estrogen dominance symptoms include PMS; insomnia; painful, lumpy breasts; headaches; anxiety.

7. Natural progesterone therapy with Prometrium, micronized compounded progesterone, or progesterone cream reverses the symptoms of estrogen dominance.

1 Speroff, L et al.   Clinical Endocrinology and Infertility 2005; p 45-57.

CHAPTER 9

THE CONTROVERSY HEATS UP: TESTOSTERONE AND WOMEN

One of the most controversial areas of BHRT is that of testosterone therapy for women. In this chapter, we're going to talk about each one of the pertinent issues in a particular order. First, we need to establish the existence of testosterone deficiency as a medical condition. Then, we will look at proof of the effectiveness and safety of testosterone treatment in women. Finally, we will look at elements of health promotion associated with testosterone therapy.

Anytime we start talking about testosterone in women, the conversation eventually turns into a discussion about sex. While it's true that when testosterone is balanced, many women rediscover their appetite for and enjoyment of sex, I believe that balanced testosterone levels have much more to do with a woman's total health and well being. And by the time you've finished reading this chapter, I hope to have convinced you of that, as well.

QUICK OVERVIEW OF TESTOSTERONE IN WOMEN

The ovaries produce 50% of a woman's testosterone; the rest is produced by the adrenal glands. Testosterone production peaks at around age 25, just like progesterone. After that, production steadily falls to the menopausal transition. Doesn't it seem logical that this would create the same imbalance with estrogen as we saw with progesterone? The end result is an increased estrogen/testosterone ratio and symptoms of testosterone deficiency.

The chart that follows should be familiar by now. It forms a large part of the rationale for consideration of BHRT.

Age Related Decline of Hormones

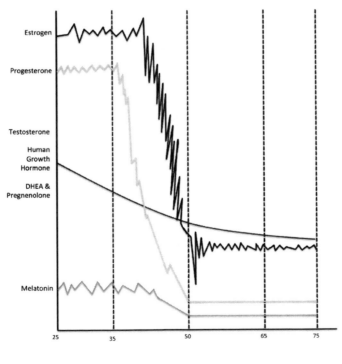

Fig. 9-1: Hormone-production decline over age

After menopause, there is no further reduction in testosterone production and, in fact, the estrogen/testosterone ratio will often normalize or even reverse as estrogen production plummets.

But remember, it's all about the ratio of a hormone to its natural antagonist, superimposed on the backdrop of the overall levels. That is why menopause is not associated with increased libido and well-being. Even though the estrogen/testosterone ratio may look better, very low levels of both don't equate with absence of symptoms. You still need to be above a critical level for each hormone to feel and function well.

Testosterone production falls by 50% between the ages of 20 and 40, and it continues to decline by 25% to menopause before it stabilizes.[4] Many people, including the critics and skeptics of BHRT, just don't see a problem with this decline. We are told it is a natural event and part of the path to increased wisdom. To this I say NONSENSE! Falling testosterone levels produce a myriad of adverse symptoms that rob women of their vitality and joy for life.

Unfortunately, the gradually declining levels of testosterone production are not the only bad news: With each pregnancy, there is a one time, non-recoverable 10-15% additional fall in testosterone production, on top of the overall decline.

In some ways, this could be seen as nature's family planning. As each pregnancy further reduces testosterone production – and lowers the resultant sex drive – it makes another pregnancy that much less likely. (And when you add in the stressors and lack of sleep that go with raising children, who says Mother Nature doesn't know what she's doing?)

The reason this is so important – and another reason every woman must be tested and treated based on her individual signs and symptoms – is that testosterone is even more highly bound to carrier proteins in the bloodstream than estrogen is. In fact, only 2% of all circulating testosterone is "free" and available to the cell for action. Meanwhile, 78% of all testosterone is strongly bound to the sex-hormone binding globulin, and SHBG has a special affinity for testosterone over estrogen.

And here's something you might not know – SHBG is dramatically increased by the use of oral estrogen.

In an excellent review, Nachtigall et al.[1] looked at the effects of various estrogens on free testosterone and found that Premarin .625 mg doubled the concentration of SHBG; Estrace (a synthetic form of estradiol) at a dose of 1 mg increased SHBG by 50%; and transdermal estrogen therapy had no effect on free testosterone. The birth control pill is an oral form of a very powerful estrogen and significantly increases SHBG. In my experience, it is very common for women on the pill to complain of reduced sex drive. The libido will always improve with discontinuation of the birth control pill.

So what does that mean to you? It means these dramatic increases in SHBG result in a drastic fall in free testosterone, which results in a lowered sense of vitality – and sex drive. This is in addition to the normal decline in testosterone production.

Some surgeries can influence testosterone levels in women. A complete hysterectomy, in which the uterus and ovaries are removed, is usually performed for serious diseases like endometriosis and results in an immediate and permanent 40% decline in testosterone production.[3,6] However, a hysterectomy with conservation of the ovaries has been shown to decrease testosterone production by 30%.[5] Damage or partial compromise to the ovarian artery at the time of surgery is believed to produce a functional impairment of ovarian testosterone production.

And here's what may be most important of all for you: We know there are clinical mechanisms that reduce testosterone production and in turn leads to symptoms. So no matter what anyone tells you, your symptoms are not all in your head!

WHAT YOU NEED TO KNOW ABOUT TESTING FOR TESTOSTERONE

A review of hormone transport in the blood is in order, because it is with testosterone that this becomes critical. Twenty percent of testosterone is weakly bound to albumin and can disassociate easily. Seventy-eight percent is strongly bound to SHBG and is not available to the cells. Only 2% is free testosterone and ready to do its job. This has important implications for how we measure testosterone in women.

I recommend measurement of free testosterone. While the test is difficult and expensive, because of the complicated lab work, it is considered the gold standard to indicate truly bio-available testosterone levels. It is worth the expense in order to get an accurate reading. Total and bio-available tests of testosterone are cheaper but not accurate. Other 'tests' add in the measurement of various binding proteins – which only serves to muddy the waters, and doesn't get us to the most basic and important issue: How much free testosterone is available to the cells so it can do the work it was meant to do?

Salivary testosterone measurements for patients NOT on replacement therapy are a reasonable method of free-testosterone assessment. For the woman already on testosterone replacement therapy, I am not in favor of using the salivary testosterone to guide effectiveness of dosing. While there is science available on the accuracy of salivary hormone levels in patients on hormone treatment, no studies have looked at the efficacy of these reported levels on a molecular basis. While it is possible that in the future, salivary levels could be used for treatment decisions, at this time I believe serum measurements are best. I believe use of salivary levels increases the chances of under treatment of patients. I have tried to use saliva measurements in this fashion and was not impressed with their accuracy in the clinical situation. The results I have achieved with serum monitoring have been outstanding and I will stick with, and recommend this approach. New evidence could change my mind, but it will take actual scientific evidence, rather than anecdotal accounts of the utility of saliva levels in patients on BHRT treatment. This should be seen as a call to action for those groups promoting saliva on-treatment measurements. The serum monitoring of hormone treatment has a long and exhaustive record. Saliva needs more work to stand on an equal basis.

To be accurate for the treatment of women, the free testosterone levels must be measured by a process called equilibrium dialysis, which is complicated but very accurate down to the picamole/liter levels at which a woman's testosterone needs to be evaluated.[2]

SYMPTOMS OF TESTOSTERONE IMBALANCE

So, we know testosterone production falls significantly from age 25 to 50. Surgery, pregnancy and hormone therapy can further reduce testosterone production and levels. It's usually at this point a skeptic would say "So what? This is a natural part of the maturation process and just another thing to deal with."

And that question is, perhaps, realistic.

But the answer depends on your perspective. In fact, I believe the real question is, or should be, "Do the declining levels of testosterone production produce symptoms that interfere with the woman's quality of life?"

In medical jargon, this set of symptoms has been labeled female androgen insufficiency and has some diagnostic criteria. Of course, there are opinions on both sides of the fence as to whether or not this syndrome is real. I believe it is, and want to give you enough information – backed up by clinical research – so you can decide for yourself.

A 2001 international consensus conference on female androgen insufficiency in Princeton, N.J., drew international experts in epidemiology, endocrinology, pharmacology, obstetrics and gynecology, urology, psychology, psychiatry and women's health. Evidence was presented and debated, which resulted in a consensus statement proposing the term "female androgen insufficiency." The consensus was that such a condition did exist and diagnostic criteria were developed and reported in a major endocrinology journal[7].

Signs and symptoms include:

- *Reduced sense of well being*
- *Depression*
- *Unexplained fatigue*
- *Changes in cognition and memory*

- *Hot flashes*
- *Reduced sex drive or libido*

Here's what is most striking about the above list of symptoms: The top four represent a large proportion of the complaints women are giving to their family doctors at this time. A large proportion of these women are in their mid-30s and 40s. This lines up with the age group experiencing declining testosterone levels. Coincidence?

The biggest problem is that, in most cases, they're not being diagnosed with female androgen insufficiency or given the appropriately directed therapy for it. Instead, they're being diagnosed with depression and are prescribed antidepressants. Depression has become the flavor of the day as a generic diagnosis for women presenting with these admittedly relatively vague complaints.

WHY IS THIS SO PREVALENT IN SPITE OF THE PROOF?

As I've stated throughout this book, the present treatment model is not only tolerated but actively promoted because it serves the powers-that-be. From a pharmaceutical perspective, depression is an indication for antidepressant therapy that could conceivably extend for years, if not a lifetime. Indeed, antidepressant sales have skyrocketed and represent a large part of the Top 10 most-prescribed drugs. Some estimates are that 20% (or more) of women over the age of 35 take an antidepressant regularly. That certainly works for the pharmaceutical companies. Antidepressant therapy requires ongoing monitoring and adjustment by a family or primary-care physician, and that is certainly easier than monitoring and adjusting hormone levels if you have never been trained to do so.

In lectures to family doctors on this topic, I have uniformly found great interest expressed about this new approach, but very few family practitioners take the next step. Learning about this area and the nuances involved is time-consuming. And many family doctors tell me that time is the one thing they do not have.

I strongly believe this easy treatment method is wrong for many of the women who take these medications for years on end. Yes, the medications allow them to cope – but not without some serious downsides. They blunt some of the joy in life. Perhaps it's just the inability of these medications to address the lack of testosterone that is the problem. And there is no question that most antidepressants significantly reduce libido, making a bad situation worse.

A large proportion of women on these medications do not like being on them, but feel they have no choice if they are to cope with life. When I see patients who are on antidepressants, one of their main goals that I hear over and over again is to take BHRT in order to get off antidepressants.

It's a realistic goal, and one that the majority is able to achieve.

The decline of testosterone is about much more than a few symptoms or a debate of hormone replacement versus antidepressants. Testosterone and the benefits that proper levels give to each woman is really all about quality of life. Life is about our relationships with others – and how we feel has a dramatic impact on them. When you're consistently sad or have a hard time finding the joy in your daily activities… when you have no energy, and feel tired all the time… when you feel as if everything is just too hard, no wonder you're depressed and aren't enjoying life.

And it's not that these women have difficult lives or no reason to be happy. In fact, most of my patients in their 40s to 60s report having an excellent relationship with their spouse or partner. They have survived the challenging years and are happy with a person who shared the journey. Unfortunately, the vast majority also report a significant reduction in their libido, which distresses them, particularly since sex allows a reconnection and maintenance of emotional intimacy with their partner.

Many of my patients tell me they still love their partner but don't care whether he shares the same bed. Most women also understand that men are emotionally simple creatures, who view sex as the external manifestation of their partners' interest and sense of connection with them. A man will commonly view his partner's lack of interest in sex as a reflection of the state of the relationship. For many, the accumulating years have moderated the need for sex, but it still remains an important way to gauge the emotional connection.

Most women know this and are upset by the effects the situation has on the happiness and satisfaction levels of their union. (Note: The above male-female dialogue can apply to same-sex relationships as well.)

TESTOSTERONE, THE DEVELOPMENT OF DISEASE, AND THE BENEFITS OF TREATMENT

Now I want to cover the third part of what I promised we'd talk about: Safety and the benefits of treatment.

The lack of testosterone is about more than lowered sexual desires or generalized feelings of depression. Not having balanced levels of testosterone is also about inflammation and an increased vulnerability to disease.

The body has many systems in place to produce inflammation to fight infection and heal injuries. As we age, science has discovered, there is a general increase in the markers of inflammation and even diseases of inflammation. In fact, there is growing evidence that more and more of the chronic diseases we can contract as we age are associated with inflammation.

Some of the most common diseases that have now been linked to inflammation might surprise you:

- *Heart disease and stroke*
- *Cancer*
- *Diabetes*
- *Arthritis*
- *Osteoporosis*
- *Alzheimer's*

One of the markers of inflammation, interleukin-6 (IL-6), is a powerful pro-inflammatory cytokine, or chemical, that is not normally detected in young healthy people. Ershler et al.[8], in an excellent review, showed that estrogen and testosterone directly reduce the production of IL-6 by blocking its transcription at the DNA in the cell. Age-related declines in estrogen and testosterone were shown to be associated with a similar inverse increase in IL-6.

Similar studies have looked at the association of progesterone and testosterone on the production of tumor necrosis factor alpha (TNF-A), another pro-inflammatory cytokine, which, when elevated, can produce much havoc in the body. The same association was seen with declines in these hormones and increases in TNF-A.

As we study more of the pro-inflammatory cytokines I believe additional associations will be proven. Treatment with the sex hormones reduces the levels of these inflammation producing compounds. The trick is in administering HRT in a safe fashion that does not produce unwanted negative effects. That is where BHRT really shines. Treatment using BHRT can be shown to reduce the levels of these damaging compounds and the diseases that are caused by them.

As you can see, BHRT is about so much more than sex! It's about improvement in the quality of life and the prevention of serious and chronic illness. This is a vital point that seems to have escaped notice of the critics. By focusing their attention and disparagement on transdermal treatments and saliva testing, they've turned a blind eye to the real benefits of replacing these hormones on physiologic levels.

The facts in the case of testosterone for women are clear: Testosterone production falls steadily in women from age 25 to menopause. This drop-off produces female androgen insufficiency, a syndrome that robs women of their quality of life in their relationships and their healthy metabolism.

Is it any wonder that as hormone levels decline, the incidence of diseases of inflammation rise and further erode quality of life?

Opposition to the safety and benefits of treatment can only be explained when the perspective of the opposing party is carefully examined.

Important Facts

1. Testosterone is an important hormone for women, just like estrogen and progesterone.

2. Testosterone levels decline 50% in women from age 20 to 40, and continue to decline to menopause.

3. Pregnancy results in a sudden and permanent 10%-15% testosterone decline that is superimposed on the natural rate of decline.

4. Oral forms of estrogen, such as the birth control pill or Premarin, can reduce free testosterone levels by 50%-70%.

5. A hysterectomy with preservation of the ovaries can reduce testosterone levels by 30%.

6. Symptoms of female androgen insufficiency include:

   - Decreased well-being

   - Depression

   - Unexplained fatigue

   - Decreased cognition and memory

   - Hot flashes

   - Reduced libido

7. Many of the symptoms of androgen insufficiency look like depression.

8. Antidepressants are commonly prescribed for the symptoms of low testosterone.

9. Testosterone has been shown to reduce the production of interleukin-6 (IL-6) and tumor necrosis factor (TNF).

10. Elevated TNF and IL-6 are associated with increased levels of inflammation.

11. Inflammation is associated with important chronic diseases such as heart disease, diabetes and cancer.

1 Nachtigall, et al.   Menopause 2000; 7(4) 243-50 / 2 Zumoff, B et al.   J Clin Endocrinol Met 1995; 80: 1429-30
3 Davis, S et al. J Endocrinol Metab 2002; 77(4): S68-71 / 4 Davison, S et al.   J Clin Endocrinol Met 2005; 90: 3847-53
5 Laughlin, G et al.   J Clin Endocrinol Met 2000; 85: 645-51 / 6 Burger, H Fert Steril 2002; 77(4): S3-4
7   Bachmann, G et al. Fertil Steril 2002; 77(4) 660-5   /   8 Ershler et al. Ann Rev Med 2000; 51: 245-70.

CHAPTER 10

HORMONES AND THE HEART

Heart disease is one of the biggest areas of concern with hormone replacement therapy for women. The discussions in previous chapters have set the stage so you have an understanding of the issues that have brought us to this place.

Your coronary arteries provide blood flow and oxygen delivery to the heart muscle. Heart attacks involve the death of a portion of the heart muscle due to occlusion (blockage) of the arteries. High cholesterol over a number of years can result in deposits on the walls of your arteries, which are already relatively narrow. Blood clots in the coronary arteries can abruptly reduce the working diameter of the artery, with a resultant significant decrease in blood flow and death of heart muscle.

A stroke involves a similar process in the arteries supplying blood flow to the brain. The only difference is a stroke damages brain tissue, rather than heart muscle.

Before menopause, women have a significantly lower chance than men of experiencing cardiovascular disease in the form of a heart attack or stroke. Both are catastrophic medical complications for the affected person and their families. But there are concrete steps you can take to reduce your risk of having a heart attack or a stroke – and HRT can help.

THE TRUTH ABOUT HRT AND YOUR HEART

In this chapter, I want to discuss the bias that women have regarding hormones and their health and to bring some usually overlooked facts into the light, so that you can make a decision about whether BHRT is right for you. To do that, you need have all the information at your fingertips.

Any time I sit down with a group of women and talk about HRT, inevitably they turn to HRT and breast cancer. However, heart disease – not breast cancer – is the major killer of women in North America.

Approximately 235,000 women die of heart attacks in the United States every year – five times the number of deaths attributed to breast cancer. The good news is, most women who have a heart attack do not die. The bad news is, many are left with permanent problems in the forms of ongoing chest pain, poor heart function and anxiety regarding their future health. Meanwhile, each year 450,000 women in the United States suffer a stroke. This is 10% more than men overall. We all are aware of the permanent disabilities that can occur in stroke survivors. These two issues are truly public health emergencies that need much more than band-aid treatment. A comprehensive preventative approach needs to be developed, and I believe BHRT should be part of that approach.

Within five years of the onset of menopause and the cessation of periods, women catch up with men in their risk of cardiovascular disease. Since the main event at this time is the drastic reduction in estrogen production, we see there must be a hormonal connection with heart disease and stroke. Of course, that does not prove that a significant drop in estrogen production causes heart disease and stroke. Reduced estrogen is just one of many hormonal changes taking place during menopause.

The irony of hormone therapy and heart disease is the circular path that popular belief has taken.

In order to really see what's going on, you have to understand the order in which the evidence accumulated. For many years, animal studies indicated that estrogen replacement therapy reduced the incidence of heart attacks and stroke. In fact, it was the accumulated weight of all this evidence that led to the idea of the Woman's Health Initiative.

Remember, the purpose of the WHI was to prove that hormone replacement in asymptomatic post-menopausal women reduced heart disease and cancer. A study by Schairer et al.[1] in 1997 followed 23,000 women for almost nine years. The researchers found that hormone replacement therapy was associated with a 23% reduction in all causes of mortality.

More important, it showed the addition of a cyclic progestin routine did not interfere with the reduction in heart disease risk seen with estrogen replacement alone. This set the stage for the WHI to extend the proof of this benefit to a larger group of post-menopausal women. Imagine the potential treatment target if proof could be obtained of a reduction in the risk of death and heart disease!

As outlined before, the biggest problem in the WHI analysis was the lack of critical thought brought to the table. The final analysis of the WHI – as it relates to cardiac protection – is well-stated in a paper by Manson et al. in the prestigious *New England Journal of Medicine*.[2] in 2003.

Their conclusion emphatically stated that estrogen plus progestin does not confer cardiac protection and may increase the risk of coronary heart disease in post-menopausal women.

The numbers were startling – a 24% increase in coronary heart disease. But no effort was made to distinguish between progestin and progesterone therapy and the risk of heart disease. It was presented as a final answer to the question and other articles were used to support the conclusion.

The Heart Estrogen/Progestin Replacement Study (HERS)[3] looked at conventional HRT in women with established heart disease. Dr. S. Hulley and associates in 1998 reported on 2,700 women with heart disease using the exact combination of Premarin and Provera used in the WHI study. These investigators found that estrogen and progestin on a daily basis had no overall effect on the risk of recurrent coronary events, or heart attacks, after an average of four years of follow-up. Remember, these are women who have already had a heart attack or who had documented heart disease. They did see an increase in the risk of blood clots and gallbladder disease.

Then there was the PHASE trial, also called the Papworth HRT Atherosclerosis Study, conducted by Dr. S.C. Clarke and associates in 2003[4], which showed no heart benefit of transdermal estradiol – with or without norethindrone (a progestin) in women with a history of heart attack. This paper supports the idea that an HRT program must be started before significant heart disease develops if it is to provide overall benefit for reducing cardiovascular disease. If atherosclerotic disease has significantly narrowed the vessels in question, neither oral nor transdermal estrogen seems to be able to decrease the chance of a second heart attack. Once the coronary vessels are affected by atherosclerotic disease, estrogen can not reverse this.

In addition, the Women's Estrogen for Stroke Trial looked at oral estradiol treatment of women who had already suffered a stroke. In this 2001 trial, Dr. C. Viscoli and associates found no overall effect on recurrent stroke and an increase in the risk of fatal stroke.[5] On the basis of this study, there is no rationale to use estrogen therapy in women who have a stroke to reduce the risk of a second stroke.

THERE'S MORE TO THE STORY

It would appear that the issue was settled for good. All the studies suggested that HRT doesn't prevent heart disease. Was this consensus valid, or is there more than meets the eye?

For example, why did the results of these studies contradict many animal and basic science studies showing the benefits of estrogen replacement therapy on coronary heart disease? A study by Dr. R.S. Kushwaha et al. in 1990[6] in baboons showed that estrogen plus progesterone directly reduced the incidence of atherosclerotic plaques, a precursor to heart disease, and these findings have been supported by numerous other studies. The findings of this study showed that estrogen therapy reduces levels of LDL (a bad cholesterol), increases HDL (a good cholesterol), and improves levels of fibrinogen. Fibrinogen is a protein produced in the liver and which circulates in the blood to assist with clotting. The higher the fibrinogen levels, the greater the risk of blood clots. Estrogen therapy also improves the function of the endothelium, which is the lining of all the blood vessels in our body. The endothelium as an organ is quite remarkable, as it has the surface area of three tennis courts! A healthy lining resists platelets sticking to the wall; platelet adhesion is one of the early events in the formation of a blood clot.Estrogen therapy also decreased lipoprotein(a), plasminogen-activator inhibitor type 1, and insulin, all of these actions reduce the risk of blood clots and vessel blockage. This study also detected adverse effects of estrogen therapy in a pill form, all of which are expected when estrogen is used in an oral form.

All of the aforementioned studies tended to look at oral estrogen and the use of a progestin, since those were the products patented and produced by the sponsoring drug company Wyeth. Are there other ways of looking at this question?

Considering the effects of the different estrogens a study by Nachtigal et al.[7] looked at the effects of different forms of estrogen on one of the hormone transport proteins made by the liver. Sex hormone binding globulin is the most important transport protein for hormones in the blood that we talked about earlier. These investigators compared Premarin, oral estradiol and transdermal estradiol as related to their effects on sex hormone binding globulin (SHBG), estradiol and estrone. Premarin increased SHBG 100%, oral estradiol increased it 45%, and transdermal estradiol had no significant effect.

This has important implications on a number of levels. Estrogen bound to SHBG is not available to the tissues for its beneficial effects. And because SHBG elevations may be associated with an increased risk of breast cancer, it should be avoided if possible. Where do you ever see mention of the increased risk of cancer secondary to the use of oral estrogen? There is also evidence that SHBG bound with estrogen has direct effects on the plasma membrane of target cells and this action may be part of the increased breast cancer risk. Only transdermal estrogen therapy effectively delivers estradiol without increasing SHBG.

This study also showed that transdermal estrogen resulted in the lowest elevation of estrone, which is an unhealthy estrogen.

So there's yet another reason to consider transdermal estrogen as the treatment of choice for estrogen replacement therapy. Why do the authorities in the area continue to turn a blind eye to this?

Another area to look at is the effect of oral versus transdermal estrogen therapy on the risk of blood clot formation. Remember that the WHI showed an increased risk of blood clots and stroke in women on Premarin and Provera. Scarabin et al.[8] conducted the ESTHER Study and first reported their results in 2003.

ESTHER stands for Estrogen and Thromboembolism Risk Study Group. The study showed that oral estrogen increased the risk of blood clots in postmenopausal women – the very same finding of the WHI! The study also showed that transdermal estrogen therapy was not associated with an increased risk of blood clots.

How many times do we need to see the same information before we develop some definite conclusions? In all the evidence I have provided, there hasn't been any to show that oral estrogen has advantages over transdermal estrogen therapy. All of the benefits we have seen are a result of transdermal therapy.

An important and often overlooked trial was the Effects of Estrogen or Estrogen/Progestin Regimes on Heart Disease Risk Factors in Postmenopausal Women (PEPI)[9]. This three-year multi-center study looked at the effect of placebo, unopposed estrogen and three estrogen/progestin regimes on selected heart disease risk factors.

The conclusion was that unopposed estrogen was most beneficial for elevating HDL (a good cholesterol). Premarin with cyclic micronized progesterone had the most favorable effect on HDL and prevented endometrial hyperplasia, a precursor to uterine cancer. It is unfortunate that Premarin pills were the estrogen choice in this study. But this was the first evidence that natural progesterone was more heart-healthy than the progestins.

I've already pointed out that progesterone and testosterone production falls from age 25 to menopause, after which progesterone production is very low and stays that way. Testosterone production stabilizes at menopause and does not fall further. So it would appear that the main hormone event at menopause is the drastic fall in estrogen secretion.

From 1980 to 2000, many medical studies showed that post-menopausal estrogen replacement decreased the risk of cardiovascular disease. Indeed, those studies led up to the WHI, whose main aim was to show that post-menopausal hormone replacement reduces the chance of heart disease and stroke.

Remember, only the Premarin and Provera arm of the WHI showed an increase in heart attack and continuous Provera seemed to completely reverse the beneficial effects of estrogen on the cardiovascular system. The Premarin-only arm of the WHI showed a 10%

reduction in the risk of heart disease, which was in complete agreement with all of the previous studies of estrogen and heart disease.

How does estrogen protect the heart? It has a number of important effects that help to reduce the incidence of heart disease and stroke.

ESTROGEN AND CHOLESTEROL

Most of us are aware that there is an association between cholesterol and heart disease. In general terms, cholesterol is a bit like a Western movie, there are good guys and bad guys. Only in this version, the bad guys often win, with the end result being a heart attack or stroke. Who are the players?

HDL – The Good Guy

Estrogen therapy increases the levels of HDL, which is the lipoprotein responsible for transporting cholesterol back to the liver for processing. Low HDL levels leave more cholesterol available for deposit into the walls of the coronary arteries. These cholesterol deposits start a chain reaction in the walls, with the end result being a reduction in the diameter of the vessel for blood flow. Therefore, we can see, the more HDL we have, the better the situation. Estrogen is on the side of the good guys!

LDL – The Bad Guy

Estrogen therapy reduces the levels of LDL cholesterol. If elevated, LDL can be deposited into the coronary vessel wall, where it starts a chain reaction that causes a fight between the body's defenses and cholesterol. Unfortunately, in a classic case of unintended consequences, the body's defenses set the stage for heart attacks and stroke. LDL deposits lead to plaque formation. Because of the heart motion, these plaques reduce vessel elasticity and increase the shear force, or internal tension in the vessel wall. These shear forces can lead to blood clots in the vessel, or plaque rupture with sudden blockage of the vessel, and death to the tissue it supplies. The end result is a heart attack with all of its negative consequences on heart muscle function.

ESTROGEN AND VESSEL RELAXATION

All major arterial blood vessels have a muscular layer in their walls. Contraction and relaxation of this muscular layer can dynamically change the vessel diameter and resultant blood flow. Wall relaxation drops blood pressure and wall constriction increases blood pressure.

Increased estrogen causes arterial vessel wall relaxation, which results in an increase in blood flow and a drop in blood pressure. Both of these effects act to reduce the chances of a heart attack or stroke. More recent studies have shown that natural progesterone and testosterone also lead to vessel dilatation via its effects on nitric oxide synthesis in the vessel wall. Perhaps there is more to testosterone than libido and sex!

Numerous studies have noted that Provera reverses the blood vessel dilation seen with estrogen therapy. (Remember, in the WHI, Premarin alone reduced heart attacks by 10%, but Premarin and Provera increased heart disease by 30 %.) I think this is much more than coincidence.

ESTROGEN AND INSULIN FOR BLOOD SUGAR REGULATION

Many studies have shown that bioidentical estrogen therapy reduces insulin levels. Insulin helps transport glucose to fat cells for storage as part of a very complicated system the body uses to keep blood sugar in a very narrow range. The narrow range of healthy blood sugar is necessary for the proper function of the brain and nervous system. Brain tissue is able to use only glucose for energy metabolism. Too little or too much has a negative effect on brain function.

As we age, we tend to gain weight, and this makes it harder for insulin to do its job. The body responds with higher insulin levels to control blood sugar. Unfortunately, high levels of insulin damage the body and contribute to accelerated aging.

Estrogen therapy, in the setting of the low levels of estrogen seen in the menopause, acts to both reduce insulin levels and reduce fasting blood sugar. Both of these effects are beneficial to the cardiovascular system, and result in a healthier body.

Proper diet and exercise are two other ways to reduce fasting glucose and insulin levels. *The Schwarzbein Principle*, by Dr. Diana Schwarzbein, is an excellent resource that illustrates in detail the effects of our dietary choices on insulin and blood glucose levels.

Some studies also have shown that certain synthetic estrogens (ethinyl estradiol and mestranol) have the opposite effects of bioidentical estrogen on blood sugar and insulin levels. The adverse effects of these two synthetic estrogens can lead to an increased risk of diabetes.

ESTROGEN AND INFLAMMATION

As you now know, inflammation leads to premature aging and can cause a predisposition to the disease process. In fact, a large number of the major diseases that people experience as they age are now associated with increased levels of inflammation. Many of the interventions used in the rapidly developing specialty of functional and regenerative medicine are directed at reducing inflammation.

C-reactive protein, a marker of inflammation, is produced in the liver and can be used to measure inflammation levels in the body. Recently, the most up-to-date cardiac risk profiles have included C-reactive protein, as it appears to be as predictive of a person's risk of heart attack as cholesterol levels.

Inflammation in the blood vessel walls reduces their flexibility and resistance to shear damage as a result of blood flow.

Oral estrogen directly increases CRP and should be avoided. That is why BHRT never includes oral estrogen therapy, and one reason the WHI, using oral synthetic estrogens, increased the risk of cardiovascular disease. Remember, with BHRT, it's all about achieving balance.

Estrogen has many positive effects on the cardiovascular system. By using transdermal estrogen in BHRT, we maximize the positive actions of estrogen therapy and minimize the negative effects on CRP production.

PROGESTERONE AND HEART PROTECTION

The story with progesterone is a bit different. Progesterone appears to have an indirect effect, through its interaction with estrogen, on cardiovascular protection.

Natural progesterone comes in two forms:

- Micronized progesterone (Prometrium capsules)

- Transdermal progesterone (progesterone cream)

I consider these two forms of progesterone to be complimentary. Each has advantages and disadvantages, and how they are used is determined by the patient's symptoms. Both of these agents have all the advantages of natural progesterone and none of the disadvantages of the progestins.

In either case, natural progesterone does not interfere with the positive effects of estrogen on cardiovascular health. The same can not be said for progestins.

One issue is that not all heart attacks in women are caused by arterial blockage; in fact, post-mortem studies of women and men who have died of heart attacks are surprising. The arteries of the men usually show a blockage that is felt to be responsible for the heart attack. But post-mortem examinations of women in the same situation show that only half of them had the same blockage.

Instead, it would appear that many fatal heart attacks in women are caused by vasospasm: The arterial wall muscle layer goes into intense spasm and restricts blood flow enough to kill heart-muscle tissue. We know that estrogen can block this wall spasm. A study in 2000 showed that progesterone, but not medroxyprogesterone acetate (MPA), enhances the beneficial effect of estrogen on vessel wall spasm secondary to exercise in women.[10]

Estrogen causes vasodilatation of the vessel wall, and natural progesterone doesn't interfere with this. This was proven in a study at the Oregon Regional Primate Research Center in 1997. Estrogen was able to prevent coronary artery vasoconstriction that occurred in response to administration of a chemical vasoconstrictor in chimpanzees. The chimp has an almost identical vessel wall to humans. However, while natural progesterone did not inhibit estrogen protection, the same was not true of Provera. Even worse, Provera actually promoted the effect of the vasoconstrictor chemical.[11]

Further proof of this concept was provided by a study comparing the effects of natural progesterone with Provera on exercise-induced myocardial ischemia (lack of oxygen delivery). The conclusion was similar to the Oregon study – natural progesterone alone is protective against heart attacks.[12]

This is not all of the evidence against Provera and its role in heart disease. The PEPI trial[9] looked at an estrogen and estrogen-progestin regime on heart disease protection[9]. The study looked at HDL, LDL and fibrinogen levels, three known risk factors for heart disease. And continuous-combined Premarin and Provera was shown to negate the positive effects of estrogen therapy.

The conclusion was that estrogen alone was the best for prevention of heart disease, estrogen and cyclic Provera was next best, and that continuous-combined was not helpful. Too bad the WHI did not know these results at the time of the study design!

As you can see, there are many levels of support for the use of natural progesterone to reduce the risk of cardiovascular disease. I am afraid the issue of the use of Provera in HRT is a closed case. There is no support for its use in a health-promotion HRT treatment program. Provera remains a good agent to be used in a cyclic fashion to regulate menstrual flow in women with lack of regular ovulation, a condition called anovulatory dysfunctional uterine bleeding that presents with irregular, heavy menstrual bleeding.

TESTOSTERONE AND HEART DISEASE

Here the situation is a bit less clear, but there appear to be some developing trends, such as discovering in the last 10 years the role of the ovaries in health promotion after menopause.

Until recently, it was common practice to remove the ovaries during hysterectomy in a woman 45 or older. Evidence is now mounting that women live longer and are healthier after menopause if their ovaries are left intact. It is now becoming usual practice to conserve the ovaries during hysterectomy up to the age of 60. Ovarian conservation in pre- and post-menopausal women supports testosterone production and results in a reduction of heart disease. Because the incidence of fatal heart disease is five times higher than fatal breast cancer in post-menopausal women, any intervention that reduces heart disease has a very large health-promotion effect. Several studies have indicated support to this concept; however, practice patterns can be slow to change.

The effects of testosterone and androstendione levels were examined in a 2001 study[13]. The thickness of the carotid artery wall can be measured by a simple ultrasound exam. The thicker the wall, the higher the degree of vessel wall atherosclerosis, or cholesterol-related damage.

These researchers found that the lower the testosterone, the thicker the carotid wall. Their conclusion was that after menopause, normal testosterone levels were associated with reduced cardiovascular disease. Similarly, a large population study in Sweden showed that reduced testosterone levels, particularly in women on HRT programs without testosterone, were associated with elevated levels of cardiovascular disease[14].

Although those findings are inconclusive – since the effects of testosterone replacement on cardiovascular disease has not been directly studied – some conclusions are apparent. The weight of the evidence leans toward a protective cardiovascular effect, summarized below. We will see in the next chapter that the relationship between testosterone and breast cancer is more straightforward.

Important Points

1. Cardiovascular disease, in the form of heart attack and stroke, is a major health risk to post-menopausal women.

2. No form of hormone replacement has been shown to be effective at reversing atherosclerotic vessel disease that is already established.

3. HRT can only be used to prevent cardiovascular disease and therefore should ideally be started in peri-menopause or with cessation of periods.

4. It is uncertain at what point beyond menopause HRT becomes ineffective to reduce risk of atherosclerosis.

5. Estrogen-replacement therapy works at a number of levels to reduce cardiovascular disease.

6. Transdermal estrogen is the most effective in this regard.

7. Natural progesterone does not block the protective effects of estrogen on the cardiovascular system and seems to have its own beneficial direct effects.

8. Progestins, and Provera in particular, block the beneficial effects of estrogen.

9. Testosterone therapy, directed at maintenance of physiologic levels, has direct benefits to the cardiovascular system.

---

1 Schairer,C et al. Epidemiology 1997; 8: 59-65 / 2 Manson,J et al. NEJM 2003; 349(6): 523-31 / 3 Grady,D JAMA 2002; 288: 49-57 4 Clarke,SC et al. BJOG 2002; 109: 1056-62 / 5 Viscoli,CM et al. NEJM 2001; 345: 1243-9 / 6 R.S.Kushwaha et al. Arteriosclerosis and Thrombosis 1991; 11: 23-31 / 7 Nachtigall,LE et al. Menopause 2000; 7: 243-50 / 8 Scarabin,P et al. The Lancet 2003; 362: 428-32 9 JAMA 1995; 273(3): 199-208 / 10 Rosano,GM et al. J Am Coll Cardiol 2000; 36: 2154-59 / 11 Raghvendra,K et al. Jour Pharmacol Exp Ther 2004; 308; 403-9 / 12 Natural medicine 1997 ;1:3, 324- 327 K Miyagawa et al / 13 Jour N Amer Meno Soc 2001 ;8; 1; 43-50 G Bernini et al. / 14 Climacteric 2007 10; 386-91 A Khatibi et al.

CHAPTER 11

HORMONES AND BREAST CANCER

In Chapter 10, we looked at cardiovascular disease in menopausal women and the effects of different hormones. Even though heart disease fatalities are five times higher than those of breast cancer, statistics don't have anything to do with the emotional issues that come with both diseases.

In my practice, I've found that whenever HRT is discussed with women, breast cancer risk as it relates to HRT is the main topic. In fact, no one has ever asked me about the reduction in risk of heart disease.

A diagnosis of breast cancer strikes at the very heart of a woman's role as a mother, a spouse and sometimes her vision of herself as a woman. The emotionality of the topic is visceral and goes beyond logic or reason.

I believe part of the problem relates to all the conflicting data around the issue of hormone therapy and breast cancer – which, just because of how contradictory and confusing it can be, leaves most women feeling frustrated and vulnerable. And without clear and concise answers to their questions, they're left with their fear alone.

The WHI clearly showed that continuous-combined HRT with Premarin and Provera increased breast cancer incidence by 30%. That was enough to cause a wholesale abandonment of HRT when the WHI was halted after the safety monitoring committee announced this news. Indeed, 50% of women who were on HRT at that time immediately discontinued using it. No one paid attention to the highlighted text in the report:

"It remains possible that (the use of) transdermal Estradiol with progesterone (not Provera) which most closely mimics the normal physiology and metabolism of endogenous sex hormones, may provide a different risk profile."

The conclusion was made to seem so simple: ***Hormones cause breast cancer.***

The problem with the WHI was that critical thinking or unbiased analysis of the results seemed to go right out the window after the announcement. No one seemed to want to ask this one very important question: *"If estrogen increases breast cancer, why did the Premarin-only arm of the study have a 23% reduction in breast cancer diagnosis?"*

But in my opinion, it's only by looking at this question that we can start to make sense of the WHI, and what it has taught us. **Premarin alone did NOT increase breast cancer.** It was only the addition of Provera to Premarin, in a continuous-combined fashion, that completely changed the risk of breast cancer.

In the years leading up to the WHI, more than 40 studies had shown that estrogen therapy alone did not increase breast cancer risk. Buried in the conclusion of the WHI Writing Group is a statement that should make all those considering bioidentical hormone therapy to sit upright and shake their heads. That statement is highlighted above.

This portion of the report was never published in the media.

I believe this is as close an endorsement of BHRT as we will see in the next few years. It is as though the pharmaceutical industry has decided to stay away from this whole area and move on to greener pastures. I will now present evidence that allows us to look a woman in the eye and tell her that BHRT is NOT associated with an increased risk of breast cancer.

ESTROGEN-ONLY THERAPY

In 1996, the American Cancer Society's research department looked at a study of more than 400,000 menopausal women. After nine years of follow-up, 1,469 breast cancers were diagnosed, and women on ERT alone had a 16% decreased risk of fatal breast cancer. At least five other studies support this line of thought. Estrogen-only therapy seems to be associated with a milder type of breast cancer.

While this study is useful to get a clearer picture of estrogen and breast cancer, beyond that, it is not helpful. Most BHRT practitioners use estrogen, progesterone and testosterone in their BHRT treatment plans, irrespective of whether the woman has had a hysterectomy. After all, as preceding sections of the book have demonstrated conclusively, it is the balance of the effects of the hormones used that produces the end result.

ESTRIOL AND ESTROGEN METABOLISM

As a proponent of combined estriol and estradiol for BHRT, I believe this is one of the missing links in this whole debate. There is no controversy over the contribution of estriol to breast health. The earlier a woman's first pregnancy is, the higher the level of estriol produced in the pregnancy, and the more pregnancies she has, the lower her lifetime risk of breast cancer.

We have already talked about a Kaiser Foundation Study that demonstrated that estriol production in pregnancy can reduce lifetime risk of breast cancer. High-estriol producers had a 58% reduction in lifetime breast cancer risk compared with low-estriol producers. And isn't it therefore plausible to think that adding estriol to a BHRT program may confer another benefit?

The findings of Kaiser Foundation Study have been confirmed by at least 10 other studies. So the question is, why is no one talking about this? Is it because you can't make enormous profits making and selling estriol, due to the patent laws? I think so!

Estriol is special among the natural estrogens because it can't be metabolized by the body into compounds that can increase breast cancer risk. Cancer reflects damage to a cell's DNA that allows the cell to grow in an uncontrolled fashion. Cancer risk appears to be directly related to the metabolism of estradiol and estrone.

In breast tissue, these two estrogens are converted into several metabolites that are collectively called catechol estrogens. See the chart on the next page.

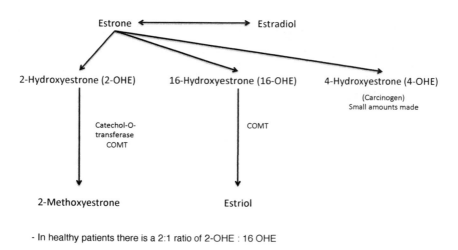

Fig. 11-1: Estrogen metabolism

The three basic types of catechol estrogens are produced as a result of the metabolism of estrone in the liver. The liver has the job of rendering these hormones inactive and placing them in a form that can be excreted. This is the process of Phase 1 and 2 detoxification we talked about earlier.

2-hydroxyestrone:

These metabolites are benign and breast-protective. The higher the level of this compound, the lower the risk of breast cancer. The use of indole-3-carbinol and DIMM can increase the production of 2-hydroxyestrone and reduce breast cancer risk. We have discussed the supplement DIMM in a previous chapter.

4-hydroxyestrone:

This metabolite reacts directly with DNA and causes mutations that can lead to abnormal growth characteristics seen with cancer.

16-hydroxyestrone:

This is a very potent estrogen metabolite that can directly induce uncontrolled cell growth. Uncontrolled cell growth is a precursor to cancer. Use of DIMM can reduce this compound's formation.

Just to make the situation even a bit more complicated is the network of protective mechanisms the body has to prevent cancer development. Chief among these is COMT (catechol 0 methyl transferase). This enzyme works to deactivate catechol estrogens into much safer methylated estrogens. Methylation of the hydroxylated estrogen metabolite is part of Phase 2 hormone metabolism or detoxification. This COMT enzyme attaches a methyl group to the estrogen metabolite making it inactive. It is possible to measure the level of COMT activity and the levels can be compared to the risk of developing breast cancer. Studies by investigators at the University of Nebraska have shown that low COMT activity is found in women with breast cancer. Methylation of the catechol estrogens allow inactivation of these aggressive compounds and expedite removal of the metabolite from the body.

Zhu et al. reported that one of the methylated estrogens normally produced in the body, 2-methoxyestradiol, has a direct action to prevent estrogen-induced cancer formation[1]. At the present time, we can't measure the levels of these metabolites in an individual. From the discussion here, the take-home points would be that all efforts to reduce estrone levels should be beneficial. Estriol can't be converted into estrone and should be considered for use in HRT. Estradiol can be converted into estrone and should be used at the lowest possible doses for relief of symptoms. When a HRT program has been finalized in a patient, the 2/16 ratio should be measured to ensure that breast cancer risk is kept as low as possible.

PROGESTERONE AND BREAST CANCER

There are numerous studies in the literature showing that a progesterone deficiency increases the risk of breast cancer.[2] These studies reported that progesterone exerts a strong protective effect, and that women with normal progesterone levels have a fivefold decrease in the risk of breast cancer. Even more astounding was the conclusion that women with progesterone deficiency, as seen with chronic infertility and anovulation, had a 10-fold increase in the risk of all types of cancer. So why should the decision of whether to use progesterone in a HRT program focus on whether the uterus is present or not? Progesterone should be part of a HRT program in ALL women to reduce the incidence or risk of breast cancer. As well, progesterone has significant brain protective effects.

As we can see, the issue of whether a woman has a uterus or not should really not enter into the decision to use progesterone in a BHRT program. It is high time to relegate the old dictum "No uterus, no progesterone" to the garbage heap in light of all the developing evidence of progesterone's health promoting effects.

The evidence is too strong to overlook the importance of progesterone. In a study on cell cultures of breast cancer, researchers showed that natural progesterone in concentrations similar to those in the third trimester of pregnancy were able to kill breast cancer cells.[3]

Meanwhile, the Million Women Study conclusively showed that the use of progestins is clearly associated with an increased risk of breast cancer[4], further corroboration of the results of the WHI and its observed increased risk with progestins. At the risk of being repetitive, there is no place for the use of progestins in any HRT program, even if synthetic estrogens are chosen. Any progestin to be considered for HRT will need exhaustive and long-run studies to prove its safety. In my opinion, this includes the raft of new progestins in development at this time. We need to study their safety profile with a jaundiced eye, rather than suffer a repeat of the MPA debacle. When we have a safe, natural compound like natural progesterone, why would we look for synthetic alternatives?

TESTOSTERONE AND BREAST CANCER

The story with natural testosterone is no different; however, until recently the proof of benefit was vague. Practitioners wanting to add testosterone to a woman's program needed to focus on the relief of low-testosterone symptoms. This area is rapidly changing, and use of testosterone for promotion of breast health is on firmer ground than ever before.

In a recent study, a group looked at the effects of adding testosterone to regular HRT programs[5]. Doing so brought the rates of breast cancer down well below those seen in the WHI and Million Women study. In fact, testosterone brought the incidence of breast cancer down to that of women who had never used hormone treatment. This is all the more significant when one realizes that these are the same HRT programs shown to increase breast cancer rates 30%. What will the studies of testosterone supplementation show in a BHRT program using estriol and natural progesterone?

Other researchers have shown in an excellent randomized, double-blinded, placebo-controlled biopsy study that testosterone inhibits breast cell proliferation induced with estrogen-progestin treatment[6].

This is one of the most powerful studies I have seen proving the benefit of testosterone treatment for breast health. The study was designed well and removes any reasons to doubt its conclusions. Indeed, the combination of these studies resulted in a compelling editorial in the *Journal of the North American Menopause Society*. The conclusion of the editorial was that the use of physiologic testosterone treatment should be added to HRT programs to promote breast health[7].

We really need to take a new look at HRT and breast cancer. Many of the conclusions of increased risk were based on poor choice of agents dictated by the sponsoring pharmaceutical companies. Self-interest in selection of agents is rampant and steered by the profit motive. HRT treatment and study deserve a much more balanced approach in selecting agents to be used. The literature is impressive when we look at the natural hormones delivered in physiologic fashion. It is time to move on!

Important Points

1. Estrogen therapy alone does not increase risk of breast cancer

2. The addition of progestins, in particular Provera, to estrogen replacement increases the risk of breast cancer.

3. Estriol is breast-protective and should be used as part of an HRT program.

4. Estrogen metabolism is complicated, but can be used to decrease breast cancer risk. Efforts to measure and increase the 2/16 hydroxyestrone ratio, if needed, are useful as part of a risk-reduction strategy.

5. Natural progesterone is breast-protective.

6. The addition of transdermal testosterone can further decrease the risk of HRT-associated breast cancer.

1 Cancer Research 1998; 58; 2269-77 B Zhu et al. / 2 AM J Epidem 1981; 114; 2; 209-17 L Cowan et al. / 3 Annals of Clinical and Lab Science 1998; 28; 6; 360-9 B Formby et al. / 4 Lancet 2003; 363; 419-27 V Beral et al. / 5 Menopause 2004; 11; 5; 531 5 C Dimitrakakis / 6 Menopause 2007; 14; 2; 183-90 M Hofling et al. / 7 Menopause 2007; 14; 2; 159-62 H Burger.

ESTROGEN THERAPY

In Chapter 7, we discussed estrogen dominance and why, in general, the vast majority of premenopausal women do not need estrogen replacement as part of a hormone-balancing program, since estrogen levels are well-maintained right up to menopause.

However, when menopause does happen, whether it's premature due to surgery or ovarian failure or natural menopause, somewhere between the ages of 48 and 54, the result is the same: A drastic reduction in circulating estrogen levels. This is when women will benefit from estrogen-replacement therapy (ERT).

Symptoms of estrogen deprivation rapidly ensue, including:

Night sweats
Painful intercourse
Decreased energy
Bladder infections
Loss of flexibility, strength and bone mass

Table 12-1 Estrogen deficiency

A woman's weight is an important modifier in estrogen dominance or deficiency. Remember, fat tissue is able to convert adrenal androgens like androstenedione into estrone, a weak estrogen. I've also mentioned that estrone and estradiol can be converted back and forth. This explains why overweight women often do not have significant hot flashes and flushes. This is why, when I consider a woman for BHRT, I always have her estradiol level measured, because it gives a basic starting point to treatment.

If her estradiol is low and the patient is symptomatic, estrogen therapy is indicated. My experience has shown that estradiol levels below 100 pmol/l(27mg/dl) are always associated with estrogen-deficiency symptoms. For me, such an estradiol level, along with the symptoms of hot flashes, night sweats, bladder infections and/or vaginal dryness, are always indications for consideration of estrogen replacement therapy. It has been mentioned before but deserves a repeat statement: There is no ideal level for a particular hormone. Hormone levels must ALWAYS be interpreted in light of the patient's symptoms, or lack of symptoms. As well, consideration must always be given to the other side of the hormone balance for the hormone in question. A good principle that I follow is that the lowest total dose of hormones needed to relieve symptoms is the goal. More is not better in BHRT.

A practitioner must make sure there are no contraindications to the use of ERT before giving a prescription.

Contraindications to ERT include:

Absolute

- Breast or uterine cancer

- Unexplained vaginal bleeding

- Pregnancy

- History of blood clots or pulmonary emboli

- Acute liver disease

Relative

- Remote history of breast, uterine or ovarian cancer

The presence of a relative contraindication should prompt a detailed discussion of the pros and cons of ERT between you and your practitioner. An absolute contraindication means the hormone should not be used until the contraindication can be removed, if possible.

Estradiol levels can be measured in blood, saliva and urine. Each of these methodologies has its own set of pros and cons. In Alberta, our health care system will provide a blood level at no cost to the patient, so it's usually my first treatment measurement of choice. Other areas of North America will have different circumstances that may change a practitioner's choice of measurement.

I recommend Biest for ERT because it can be prepared in almost any ratio of estriol to estradiol. I prefer the 80/20 preparation, but I know many knowledgeable practitioners who use 50/50 or 90/10, so if your doctor or provider uses something different, it's nothing to worry about – your results are what counts.

I have mentioned numerous reasons for not using estrogen by mouth, but I believe it's an issue that's important enough to be mentioned again. The problems with oral or pill forms of estrogen include:

- Increase in sex hormone binding globulin (SHBG), which has a special affinity for testosterone and can worsen symptoms of androgen insufficiency syndrome. (Why choose a route of delivery that worsens another part of the patient's hormone imbalance?)

- Increased levels of C-reactive protein (CRP), which is a marker of inflammation. Since I believe BHRT is one element of an anti-aging program, any increase in inflammation is to be avoided. Remember, inflammation is now recognized as an important causative agent in many of the important ailments we are prone to, including cancer, heart disease, Alzheimer's disease and diabetes.

- Increased risk of blood clots as seen in the WHI. Oral estrogen increases levels of fibrinogen, which makes the blood stickier.

From now on, when we talk about estrogen therapy, I will always be referring to transdermal therapy.

In addition to relief of the above list of complaints, estrogen has a number of health promotion effects. They include:

BRAIN FUNCTION

Estrogen has been shown to increase the flow of blood to the brain. It also stimulates the development of brain cell connections with improvements in memory. In addition, we know estrogen slows the breakdown of serotonin, dopamine and nor-epinephrine – neurotransmitters that help mood and cognitive abilities.

Many studies show that estrogen appears to reduce the risk of Alzheimer's disease. The effects of ERT in this area seem to be most noticeable when it is started soon after the onset of the menopause. A reduction in Alzheimer's was not seen with the WHI. Studies have shown that Provera can prevent many of the beneficial effects of estrogen in the brain. Perhaps this is another unintended negative consequence to the decision to use it for profit motive despite evidence of problems with it at the time of WHI study design.

Because estrogen improves many aspects of cognitive function, it should be considered as part of a preventative health program in a newly menopausal woman.

There is no question that ERT improves sleep in a symptomatic woman with hot flashes. The brain's restorative and repair processes take place during sleep, so this is how ERT is able to optimize brain function. I believe we are not far away from routine measurements of brain-derived neurotropic factor, and that studies with BHRT will show significant improvements in this vital brain-repair compound.

OSTEOPOROSIS

Bone density reaches its peak in the early 20s and then begins a gradual decline. With menopause comes an acceleration of bone-density loss, and this has become a major public health issue as people continue to live longer than ever before.

One effect of the WHI was a wholesale reduction in the use of HRT – which is a tragedy, because there is no other treatment today that's been proven to be as effective in the prevention and treatment of osteoarthritis as a well-designed hormone replacement program.

All three of the sex hormones have receptors in bone, and their net effect is to preserve bone density.

Estrogen seems to prevent bone loss primarily by modulating the activity of osteoclasts, the bone cells responsible for bone breakdown. Bone is a very dynamic tissue with a continued fight between the forces that build it up and tear it down. Estrogen reduces breakdown, while progesterone and testosterone help to build new bone. A balanced BHRT program helps bone density stay in a range that avoids fractures.

OSTEOARTHRITIS

This is the arthritis of old age or wear-and-tear on the body. Studies show that ERT significantly reduces the risk of developing osteoporosis. Even the follow-up WHI studies on the Premarin-only group showed a reduced need for joint replacement.

Low levels of circulating estradiol were equated with a doubling of the risk of knee osteoarthritis.

COLON CANCER

Did you know that colon cancer is the third-leading cause of cancer death in women? It's one of the most treatable cancers when caught early enough. However, we also know – and even evidence from the WHI study confirmed – that ERT can reduce a woman's risk of colon cancer by up to 50%.

Although how this works isn't completely understood, promising research shows that the effect of estrogen on the action of bile acids in the colon makes the difference.

Now that you've got a better understanding of the advantages to ERT, let's go over the different options for ERT in a BHRT program.

TRANSDERMAL BIEST

Because of the advantages of estriol against breast cancer, I favor the use of Biest for ERT. There are many pharmaceutical transdermal estradiol patches and gels, but none contains estriol. They are bioidentical, but none can hold a candle to Biest. In addition, a compounding pharmacy can add testosterone to Biest, allowing the practitioner to kill two birds with one stone.

I have prescribed Biest for a number of years and feel that application to the vulva is the most effective. Absorption there is excellent and predictable. With an 80/20 formulation, 0.5-2.0 mg in .25cc of HRT cream seems to be a good starting place. Please be aware that doses in BHRT are subject to great variation regarding dosage. Choice of product, cream base selection and area of application all are important factors. While I give some guidance, your BHRT practitioner should be trusted to guide your therapy.

The chart that follows is used to illustrate the rationale for this starting dose. Previous studies using a 50 mcg/day estradiol patch demonstrated that even this dose of estrogen was sufficient to improve bone density.

Previously I mentioned that the estrogen receptor is a dimer. That means two molecules of estrogen must bind to the receptor to initiate a change in shape of the receptor that allows it to bind to DNA. Remember, the different estrogens have different affinities for the receptor and different strengths of action at the DNA level. A 2.0 mg dose of 80/20 Biest product gives a close estimate of a 50 mcg/day dose of estradiol alone. However, this gives us all the advantages of a significant amount of estriol with its breast-protection benefits.

Different Biest ratios would necessitate a change in dosage to ensure that the proper amount of estradiol is present. For example, if the 50/50 Biest were used, the dose would have to be reduced to avoid too much estradiol in the prescription. The chart is busy, but it does show there is science behind the choice of dose for this particular product. At this time I favor the 80/20 ratio to optimize estriol activity. This decision may change as a result of research I am conducting at this time.

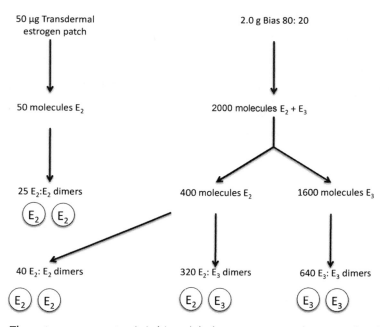

The estrogen receptor is is bimodal, the receptor needs two molecules of estrogen to have a DNA response.

Fig. 12-1: Estrogen metabolism

I ask my compounding pharmacy to put this dose of Biest in .25 cc of cream to allow easy application in the morning after a bath or shower. After a couple hours there is no worry about loss of product with urination. Some women will find it more convenient to apply the cream in the evening or before bed. However, using Biest in the morning minimizes the chance of having it come in contact with your male partner – most men have enough environmental estrogen exposure as it stands. In the end, there is no ideal time; the best is the one that encourages regular use of the cream.

I initially used a transdermal route, having the patient apply it to another area of the skin, but discovered that absorption was variable and the patient had to come into my office multiple times for testing. An unintended benefit of vulvar Biest application has to do with urinary incontinence. Loss of urine with laughing, coughing, sneezing and jumping is common in post-menopausal women. Approximately 50% of these women will have significant improvement in this unpleasant problem with use of vaginal estrogen. As well, there are good studies supporting a role for estriol in promoting an increase in collagen at site application. Since the urine incontinence is the result of collagen loss and structural changes as a result of childbirth, application of Biest to the vulva cannot hurt. In addition, use of estrogen on the vulva always improves vaginal dryness with sex, which is a very common complaint in post-menopausal women

A secondary benefit of vulvar application is that if testosterone is added to the Biest, it doesn't result in increased growth of dark hair. Whenever you apply testosterone to skin that has hair follicles, the hormone will cause the hair to become more noticeable and dense. (I can tell you that hell hath no fury like a woman whose arm hair coarsens and darkens.) The outside vaginal lips have no hair follicles and therefore hair growth is not a problem when a testosterone con- taining cream is used there.

Another advantage of BHRT involves treatment monitoring. Because Biest contains estradiol, it is possible to monitor treatment levels and adjust the dosage when needed. In order to accurately measure estradiol levels, I ask my patients to switch their applica- tions to bedtime for three days before the blood test, because Biest is very effectively absorbed and levels spike quite high several hours after application. When the blood test is done the next morning, a 10- to-12-hour post-application level results. This appears to be very reproducible and allows for reasonable treatment decisions.

This is certainly an improvement on traditional HRT, as synthetic hormones do not show up on assays for estradiol, and for this reason traditional HRT has never used blood levels to guide treatment. This means that BHRT allows a much more precise replacement of hormones than a simple symptom score allows. An estradiol level of 100 pmol/l(27 mg/dl) or more, 12 hours post-application, reliably results in the loss of hot flashes.

My target blood level for estrogen replacement is 150 pmol/l(40 mg/dl) of estradiol. I usually wait eight weeks after a dose change to order a blood measurement, because by this time a new equilibrium has been established in the patient. Remember, hormones take a while to reach a steady state in the body. Eventually, a new hormone dose is incorporated into fat stores in the body. This is why skipping a day of hormone application doesn't result in any increase in symptoms. The body just borrows some of the hormone stored in fat cells for general use. In fact, discontinuation of hormone creams will not show up as symptoms for three to four weeks as the body uses up the stored hormone in fat tissue. The more fat, the more stored hormone. The patient is seen four to six weeks after the blood test and a symptom chart is used to track patient responses and compare them to the blood levels. The correlation of hormone levels to the patient's symptoms is critical and cannot be over emphasized. Without constant reference back to the patient, the process of BHRT is flawed and inferior results will be obtained. This is also the Achilles heel of BHRT – namely, in order to do this area well you have to spend time with the patient. BHRT will not work with a five-minute appointment. BHRT is truly ALL about the patient, an individualized treatment for a one-of-a-kind person. When patients finally get this, resistance to proper compensation for the practitioner abates.

A good correlation is seen between symptom resolution and blood levels in most cases. If the symptoms do not resolve with adequate blood levels, then the possibility of adrenal fatigue or stress becomes more likely, which helps us to further diagnose and treat symptoms.

Once an ERT program is stable, I suggest the patient take a 24-hour urine test for hormones. This test lets us analyze the estrogen quotient (estriol/estradiol plus estrone), which can be used to assess risk of breast cancer on treatment. An EQ of 1.0 or greater equates with a reduced risk of breast cancer and seems to be always achievable with the use of Biest 80/20.

The 24-hour urine test also measures the 2/16 hydroxyestrone ratio, which should be greater than 1.0 for a reduced risk of breast cancer. If the ratio is less than 1.0, DIMM or I3C can be used to increase 2-hydroxylation and improve the ratio. After this testing, the post-menopausal woman will need to be evaluated yearly with a simple blood test. I don't recommend repeat urine testing unless a problem was identified and a repeat urine test is needed to ensure correction of the problem.

A number of private labs in the United States perform this 24-hour urine test. I've found Meridian Valley in the Seattle area offers excellent quality and very good practitioner support in the United States. Here in Canada, Rocky Mountain Labs in Calgary is able to provide our patients this service.

ESTRADIOL PELLETS

Compounding pharmacies can make estradiol, progesterone and testosterone pellets for insertion under the skin. This is a very convenient method of hormone replacement, since a pellet will generally last four to six months after insertion. I do not have much experience with this option, as these are not readily available in my area of Canada and are quite expensive. Many compounding pharmacies in the United States can make pellets affordably.

ESTRADIOL PATCHES

A variety of pharmaceutical estradiol patches are available. They have the advantage of considerable science behind the characteristics of their estradiol absorption and blood levels. However, a major limitation in their use is the inability to combine testosterone therapy. And none of them have estriol. However, they are well-tolerated, effective and of reasonable cost. And, of course, they are bioidentical with all the advantages that go with BHRT.

DURATION OF USE

Probably one of the most common questions patients ask when they start feeling better is, "How long do I need to stay on BHRT?"

My answer is always the same: "For as long as you want to feel the way you do now."

We have no way to restart normal ovarian function after the onset of menopause. Unless and until we do, I believe BHRT is a cornerstone of a longevity program that aims to put more life in your years instead of just more years in your life. And I believe that much more will be available on this topic in the years to come.

Important Points

1. Estrogen production declines significantly at the time of menopause and with surgical removal of the ovaries.

2. Symptoms of estrogen deprivation include:

    - Night sweats
    - Dry and painful intercourse
    - Decreased energy
    - Frequent bladder infections
    - Loss of flexibility and strength
    - Decreased bone density

3. Estrogen levels should be measured when estrogen treatment is contemplated.

4. Blood, saliva or urine measurement can be used at the start of therapy.

5. Absolute contraindications to ERT include:

    - Existing breast or uterine cancer
    - Unexplained vaginal bleeding
    - Pregnancy
    - History of blood clots
    - Acute liver disease

6. Avoid oral estrogen replacement therapy as it increases C-reactive protein, blood clotting proteins and sex hormone binding globulin.

7. Estrogen therapy is associated with:

    - Improved brain function
    - Decreased loss of bone density and possibly increased bone density
    - Reduced osteoarthritis symptoms
    - Reduced chances of colon cancer

8. I prefer Biest, applied daily to the vaginal lips, or vulva with or without testosterone.

9. The target for serum estradiol level is150 pmol/l(40 mg/dl) when measured 10-12 hours after Biest application.

10. Consider doing a 24-hour urine hormone measurement when therapy goals have been reached. Estrogen quotient and 2/16 ratios can be measured in the test and modified to reduce chances of breast cancer.

CHAPTER 13

PROGESTERONE THERAPY

In Chapter 8, we discussed the important facts about progesterone. Briefly:

Progesterone is the natural antagonist to the growth-inducing effects of estrogen. Every month a premenopausal woman's body provides a 10-day dose of progesterone after ovulation to mature the lining of the uterus and prepare it for menstruation. Regular periods are the result and continue to be an indicator of good health.

Progesterone production falls dramatically – by a factor of at least 50% – from age 25 to 40. Estrogen production, on the other hand, is well-maintained over this time, and is, in fact, even increased due to weight gain and environmental exposure to xenoestrogens.

This estrogen dominance is the single-most common condition that I see in premenopausal women. And yet, in conventional modern gynecology, this is an almost unknown condition – in fact, I myself was unaware of it until a few short years ago. I've gone to many medical conferences over the years and no one was talking about estrogen dominance to gynecologists. In fact, it was only with exposure to bioidentical hormone ideas that I came to see its existence.

Now in my regular gynecology practice, I see a veritable avalanche of estrogen dominance, with symptoms such as:

Premenstrual syndrome	Heavy menstruation
Painful, lumpy breasts	Insomnia
Anxiety	Unexplained weight gain
Depression	Foggy thinking
Fluid retention	Decreased sex drive

Table 13-1: Estrogen dominance

It's an impressive list, and if one looked for these complaints in a busy family practice, they would be seen in a large number of patients.

There seems to be no end to the underlying causes of this epidemic. Much has been said about the compromises to our food supply. What works well for the food manufacturers does not normally serve the public interest, though I see encouraging signs that this will change over time.

Organic food sections in the ordinary supermarket are growing rapidly here in Canada. Consumers are voting with their pocketbooks and the grocery stores are listening. The grocers in turn put pressure on the food growers to provide them with healthy alternatives to the regular choices. Governments are helping by designing and enforcing standards for organic foods. The consumer wants – and deserves – confidence that the extra cost of organic foods is reflected in products that actually lack pesticides, antibiotics and growth agents.

It is a slow process that will continue to gain momentum as the average person starts to take back control of some elements of his/her life. Yes, it's expensive to eat healthy, but I hope, over time, that differential will lessen. Unfortunately, as it stands now, the less-advantaged people are the ones most affected by our compromised food supply and the ones least able to bear its cost.

For the time being, we will still have to deal with the epidemic of estrogen dominance. And the first-line treatment is progesterone. Of course, when I say progesterone, I mean natural progesterone. This chapter will refer to natural progesterone in all its different forms.

As I have mentioned before, the whole idea of estrogen dominance was introduced and championed by Dr. John Lee. It is very easy to discuss these issues now, but Dr. Lee started to voice his concerns well before the WHI and its results were available. His ideas were correct and have stood the test of time. It's a pity Wyeth did not consider him as a consultant for the initial design of the WHI. I can't help thinking the HRT world would look a lot different today if that had been the case. It takes a special degree of courage to stand up against the powerful authorities in the medical community and tell them they are wrong.

We owe a debt of gratitude to Dr. Lee, and lost one of the great pioneers in the area of BHRT with his death in 2003. You can read about his ideas in his books, such as *What Your Doctor May Not Tell You About Menopause: The Breakthrough Book on Natural Hormone Balance*, written with Virginia Hopkins, and *What Your Doctor May Not Tell You About Pre-menopause: Balance Your Hormones and Your Life From Thirty to Fifty*, written with Dr. Jesse Hanley and Hopkins. All of BHRT has been built on the foundation Dr. Lee provided. While I may not completely agree with all of his ideas, they certainly are a good start to developing a full BHRT program. The biggest contribution he made was in advancing natural progesterone as the great balancer and protector to the effects of estrogen in the body.

THE BIRTH CONTROL PILL AND ITS PROBLEMS

If a woman has heavy periods because of estrogen dominance, the easiest and safest thing to do is to replace the hormone she is deficient in. Natural progesterone is the best antidote to estrogen dominance and the first-line treatment. Unfortunately, modern gynecology often resorts to the birth control pill. And while it's true that the pill can control the symptoms, it magnifies the underlying factors creating the problem.

The pill is a combination of powerful estrogens and progestins. Since its development, it has constantly changed with an overall view to reducing the dose of hormone amounts. In fact, modern low-dose oral contraceptives have a fraction of the estrogen and progestins that the early pills had. Despite this reduction, the current low-dose pill still represents a tremendous hormone load on the body.

For contraception, the pill has very few competitors and a number of advantages. A sexually active young woman needs a reliable, convenient method of contraception and the pill fits the bill. Her progesterone production is at its peak, and, for a variety of reasons that have not been worked out, she is most likely to tolerate the possible adverse effects of the pill without consequence. However, as this woman ages, her ability to tolerate the pill wanes, perhaps because of a decline in hormone metabolism capacity.

The birth control pill represents a tremendous estrogen load to the body. It has to! It shuts down normal ovulation and estrogen production as it prevents pregnancy. As well, a high level of estrogen is needed to prevent irregular or breakthrough bleeding during the cycle. In fact, the total estrogen dose in the pill over a month is at least four times the normal female production. This dose of estrogen allows the pill to do its job. The estrogen in the birth control pill is ethinyl estradiol (a modified estrogen) and doesn't show up on blood tests. In fact, when you measure estradiol levels in a young woman on the pill, they are in the menopausal range. Despite this, her estrogen load is at least four times normal. The birth control pill also has a significant amount of a progestin to balance the high levels of estrogen. The balance is heavily weighted toward the progestin side of the equation. This helps prevent sperm from getting to the egg that lies in wait in the fallopian tube after ovulation. As well, with a progestin dominance, the birth control pill will usually give a woman lighter than normal periods. Light periods are desirable and another reason the birth control pill continues to be popular. At this time there is no bioidentical option to the pill.

While progestins work at the level of the uterine lining to counteract synthetic estrogens, the progestins do not mimic the actions of progesterone in the brain. It is a common observation that as women age, their ability to tolerate the pill diminishes. They will commonly tell you that they took the pill in their 20s without side effects, but noticed they felt unwell on the pill in their 40s. The side effects often cited are anxiety, weight gain and bloating. Not exactly a surprise, considering the high dose of estrogen in the birth control pill.

I believe this is because of estrogen dominance. Due to its high estrogen load, the pill worsens this situation. The progestins in the pill are unable to work the same as natural progesterone in the brain and side effects increase.

It's not all bad – the young women who most need the contraceptive benefit of the pill are the ones most able to tolerate it. This doesn't apply to the women with heavy menstrual bleeding. Estrogen dominance causes extra growth of the uterine lining, which, when shed, creates painful and heavy periods, or menorrhagia. The menstrual cycle and periods are still regular, but the monthly bleeding is heavy and prolonged, with blood clots and accidents a regular occurrence. Having an accident in public, when the heavy flow overcomes the protection, is not tolerable to most women.

As long as the cycle is regular, which is indicative of regular ovulation, natural progesterone is the ideal compound to correct the problem. It doesn't increase the estrogen load to the body and dramatic improvements are often seen in the form of less anxiety and better sleep, as well as a reduction in menstrual flow. The heavy period is a clue to the presence of estrogen dominance. This is why gynecologic procedures to correct the heavy flow don't always leave the woman with a dramatically better life. In fact, the use of progesterone in this setting dramatically reduces the need for any type of surgery, which would not be favored by surgeons whose livelihood depends on a regular, full patient list.

TREATING HEAVY BLEEDING

Another problem commonly seen in women in their 40s is irregular and/or heavy bleeding, called menometorrhagia or anovulatory dysfunctional uterine bleeding. This reflects loss of regular ovulation and uncontrolled endometrial growth, which, if not corrected, it can lead to endometrial hyperplasia, a precursor to uterine cancer.

Even though estrogen dominance is one of the contributing factors, natural progesterone has not been helpful for treating this condition. I have tried continuous and cyclic forms of natural progesterone therapy with poor success. The pill is effective, but exacerbates estrogen dominance.

Our old enemy, Provera, has a place in the treatment of this condition, much to my surprise! When given at a dose of 10-20 mg per day for the first 12 to 14 days of the cycle, Provera will quite reliably restore regular menstruation without significant side effects. But if brain symptoms of estrogen dominance persist, a small amount of natural progesterone cream will provide the solution.

This just goes to show it's important not to throw the baby out with the bathwater. Cyclic Provera doesn't reverse the benefits of estrogen on the heart, and can correct a problem that otherwise will require surgery. But for the typical premenopausal woman with estrogen dominance, natural progesterone is the antidote for her problems.

Also, natural progesterone is an integral part of a post-menopausal woman's hormone replacement program.

The rest of this chapter will look at the options of natural progesterone replacement. One issue is cyclic versus continuous treatment. If progesterone is given in a continuous fashion with no breaks, receptor down-regulation may occur. The body senses too much progesterone for too long and protective mechanisms are deployed.

Too much progesterone in either quantity or duration causes the progesterone receptors to become less sensitive to the presence of progesterone. Research has shown that as few as five days without progesterone per month will prevent receptor down-regulation.

This makes sense when we consider various scenarios. If given in a cyclic fashion, progesterone will usually create a menstrual cycle if there is sufficient estrogen priming of the uterine lining. This is not a problem for the premenopausal-cycling women who expects a monthly period. All she has to do is skip the progesterone treatment for the days she menstruates. I have found most premenstrual, estrogen-dominant women feel best if they take their progesterone through the month on the days they don't bleed.

It is possible to use different combinations of duration and dose during the month. Some practitioners like to vary the dose of progesterone during the cycle to mimic the natural body rhythm. This involves a low dose of progesterone in the first half of the cycle and a higher dose in the second half. I understand the rationale and if it works well for them and their patients, carry on. I am a "keep it simple, stupid" person, and find the same dose every day where no bleeding occurs to work well. This is not cast in stone. The situation is different for post-menopausal women who have finished their periods. Most of them do not want their menses to resume, and we will do our best to heed these wishes.

In fact, this is why the WHI chose a continuous progestin approach despite the absence of proof of safety at the time of study design. Obviously the decision did not work in the study's favor, but we would do well to heed the reasons behind the decision.

No BHRT program will work if you can't get the patient to follow the program. Most post-menopausal women do not want to resume their periods and we need to listen! As well, treatment will work best if progesterone receptor down-regulation can be avoided. A simple and effective way to satisfy both concerns is to skip all prescribed hormones on Sundays. On average, the patients gets four to five hormone-treatment-free days every month and no periods. It's best of both worlds! If bleeding occurs, it is a tip-off that the estrogen dose is too high.

I aim for the lowest dose of estrogen I can use to rid the patients of their estrogen-deprivation symptoms. I monitor blood tests to ensure I have hit my target range and find that very rarely do they have to cope with unwanted bleeding.

Some women will feel better using progesterone every day. I have been unable to find a problem with this in the hormone literature and feel it is a safe approach. It does make me slightly nervous, from a receptor down-regulation point of view, but it works for them. Time will tell on this topic.

Earlier, I mentioned checking blood levels to monitor estrogen treatment. The situation is different for progesterone. I do measure progesterone on treatment to give me an idea of estrogen/progesterone balance, but do not find the absolute values to be of assistance. All women on Prometrium will have levels equal to or above a mid-luteal-phase progesterone level, which is 15 mmol/l. Progesterone cream creates much lower levels than the oral form. This seems to have more to do with the transport mechanism for a transdermally applied progesterone, and the lower blood levels do NOT equate with a loss of effectiveness in preventing endometrial hyperplasia.

Progesterone can be taken in an oral form or applied as a cream. Each has advantages and disadvantages. In some patients, I use a combination to minimize that woman's list of symptoms. There is no right or wrong, no better or worse, just two great choices to be used as needed.

PROGESTERONE CAPSULES (PROMETRIUM, OR MICRONIZED PROGESTERONE)

Regular progesterone taken by mouth is inactivated by stomach acid and will not work. A process called micronization gets around this problem. Progesterone is placed in small microsomes that are resistant to stomach acid. Once in the small intestine, the microsomes break down from the action of digestive enzymes and the progesterone is absorbed. From there, it travels to the liver, where a large percentage of it is metabolized. Because of this metabolism in the liver, oral doses of progesterone can be five to 10 times the transdermal dose. There does not seem to be an adverse effect of the higher dose of progesterone being presented to the liver, and perhaps there are some advantages.

In particular, we don't see the induction of binding and clotting protein proteins that occurs when estrogen is given orally. However, liver metabolism does produce a compound called 5-allopregnenolone that has one great benefit: It is a natural sleep-inducing agent. Most estrogen-dominant women sleep poorly. Micronized progesterone is the cure for what ails them: 100-200 milligrams of Prometrium, or micronized progesterone (made by a compounding pharmacy), will restore sleep to normal. I have seen this over and over again. I do not often go above 200 mg, as I think you can get too much of a good thing. If more progesterone is needed for symptom relief, the addition of 20-40 mg of progesterone cream will do the trick.

Prometrium is packaged in a capsule with peanut oil to aid absorption. If a patient has peanut allergies, compounded micronized progesterone can be used safely. Progesterone capsules are the form I most commonly use. Use of a compounded progesterone allows the addition of melatonin 3-9 mg to the capsule, for women with sleep problems that are resistant to progesterone alone. They are simple, effective and free of side effects. Improve a women's sleep and you do the whole family a favor!

Prometrium is produced by the pharmaceutical company Solvay and can be obtained by prescription at any pharmacy. Micronized compounded progesterone is formulated by a compounding pharmacy.

Occasionally, a woman will report that her sleep is worsened by oral progesterone. There is a small subset of women who metabolize progesterone in a slightly different fashion. It would appear that they make deoxy-corticosterone from the progesterone, which can be activating rather than sedating. A simple switch to progesterone cream will solve this problem.

TRANSDERMAL PROGESTERONE CREAM

This is as good as orally administered progesterone and I use it frequently. I do not recommend the over-the-counter creams; instead, I suggest compounded progesterone cream from a compounding pharmacy. This way, you can ensure the quality, dosage and proper base cream to be used. I will have more to say about compounding pharmacies in Chapter 16. I would stay away from any cream containing "natural" progesterone. Testing has shown that up to half of these products did not contain progesterone! If it's not in there, it's not going to help you!

I suggest the use of progesterone cream twice daily, as it is rapidly metabolized in the body. Typical doses for my patients are 10-40 mg, twice daily. I know of practitioners who use much higher doses without apparent ill effects. One of my mottos has always been to use the least amount of a medication to do the job. With higher doses, we just need to be aware that we are using progesterone as a drug, not as a physiologic hormone replacement program.

One of the big issues with progesterone cream is the lack of target-range blood levels with its use. Conventional medicine has long argued that transdermal progesterone doesn't produce serum progesterone levels required to guarantee safety of the uterine lining. Remember, estrogen increases endometrial growth and progesterone combats the estrogen effect. I completely agree with this observation after monitoring blood levels of hundreds of patients using it. It appears that the transport mechanism for progesterone cream is different than that of estrogen and testosterone, because the red blood cells can take up huge quantities of progesterone as they traverse the capillary bed of the skin where the cream was applied.

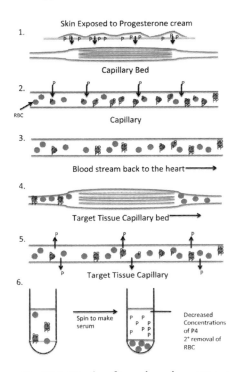

Fig. 13-1: Uptake of transdermal progesterone

The delivery to the target organs – brain, uterus, breast and blood vessels – occurs very efficiently. That's because as these hormone-laden blood cells go through the capillary beds of the target tissues, the hormones on the surface of the red blood cells are "wiped" off and head to their target cells in that tissue.

Progesterone bound to red blood cells doesn't raise serum levels very much, as the RBCs are removed from the serum before the hormone level is run. Dr. George Gillson and Tracy Marsden, in their excellent book, *You've Hit Menopause, Now What?*, go over this issue in great detail for those with an interest in this area. The end result of progesterone cream use is low serum levels and concerns by conventional doctors that this method of progesterone administration is ineffective for protection of the uterine lining. As is often the case in this area, things are never as simple as they would seem. I agree with their concerns, but will try to show how safety can still be preserved with low serum levels.

We know from saliva testing of hormones that there is very efficient delivery of progesterone with use of the creams. As well, patient symptom relief is excellent.

In the medical community, hormone delivery using progesterone cream is a very emotional subject. There is no question that serum progesterone levels do not rise into the luteal phase zone with the use of cream. However, there is good evidence that endometrial delivery is sufficient to ensure prevention of endometrial hyperplasia.

Helene Leonetti et al. compared topical progesterone cream at a dose of 40 mg twice daily with Provera 10 mg per day in patients getting Premarin .625 mg per day[1]. An endometrial biopsy was done before and after treatment to look for endometrial hyperplasia. There was no difference in the effects of the two regimes, although most of the patients preferred the progesterone cream.

Another point in favor of progesterone cream was a study comparing Prometrium 200 mg per day with progesterone cream 40 mg per day[2]. When whole blood was used to measure hormone content, no difference was seen with the progesterone levels of these two approaches.

Numerous other studies have shown beyond a shadow of a doubt that topical progesterone provides adequate endometrial protection despite low serum levels[3,4,5,6]. Progesterone cream can be applied anywhere on the body. It is often best to rotate sites, to spread out the fat tissues exposed to the progesterone, but there are no restrictions as to where to put it. There is no proof that site rotation is needed, this is just my preference.

If luteal-phase breast tenderness is an issue, why not apply it to the breasts at this time of the cycle to counteract the effects of estrogen? Some evidence suggests the cream reduces wrinkles. Why not use it sparingly on the face one or two or times per cycle?

The only issue that differentiates the cream from oral progesterone is conversion. Remember, when we looked at the sex steroid synthesis chart, progesterone was at the top. Transdermal progesterone can be converted into estrogen and testosterone, while the oral forms of progesterone can't be converted to the other hormones. This is especially important in women with estrogen dominance, as you don't want to increase their estrogen load. For those women, I always suggest oral progesterone, quite the opposite stance from estrogen. In hormones as in clothes, one size doesn't fit all! Follow-up testing of all sex hormone levels should be done in patients starting progesterone cream treatment.

VAGINAL CREAM/ORAL DROPS OR LOZENGES

I have little experience with these options and see no benefit to them. If you are using these methods and they work for you, stick with them. New patients should consider capsules or cream.

Important Points

1. Regular periods in a premenopausal woman are a good indicator of health and reflect monthly progesterone production that counteracts the proliferative actions of estrogen.

2. Progesterone production falls at least 50% from age 30 to 50.

3. Estrogen production often rises from age 30 to 50 due to

   - Weight gain
   - Xenoestrogens exposure

4. These changes in estrogen production relative to progesterone production create estrogen dominance, a condition coined by Dr. John Lee.

5. Symptoms of estrogen dominance include:

   - Insomnia
   - Painful, tender breasts
   - PMS
   - Weight gain
   - Heavy menstruation
   - Depression
   - Foggy thinking
   - Decreased sex drive

6. The birth control pill can worsen symptoms of estrogen dominance.

7. Irregular, heavy menstrual bleeding is best treated with cyclic Provera.

8. Natural progesterone is the best therapy for symptoms of estrogen dominance.

9. Oral progesterone Prometrium or micronized progesterone at bedtime restores healthy sleep to most women with insomnia.

10. Both oral and transdermal progesterone therapies are effective and can be used together.

11. Serum progesterone levels are not helpful when transdermal progesterone is used.

12. Post-menopausal women can skip HRT on Sundays and still not have the resumption of periods.

13. Premenopausal women are advised to not use HRT when they are menstruating.

14. Sex hormone levels should be checked on all patients starting progesterone cream treatment to ensure that significant conversion to estrogen and testosterone doesn't occur.

1 Alternative Therapies 2005; 11; 6; 36-8 H Leonetti et al. / 2 J Clin Pharmacol 2005; 45; 614-9 A Hermann et al. / 3 Menopause 2005; 12; 2; 232-7 F Stanczyk et al. / 4 Climacteric 2000; 3; 155-60 B Wren et al. / 5 Fertil Steril 2003; 79; 1; 221-2 H Leonetti et al. / 6 Maturitas 2002; 41; 1-6 J Lewis et al.

CHAPTER 14

TESTOSTERONE THERAPY IN WOMEN

In Chapter 9, we looked at the evidence of androgen deficiency syndrome. Its symptoms are subtle and easily overlooked. Remember, testosterone production falls from a peak at age 25 (when the libido is in high gear) right through to menopause. And we've also talked about how each pregnancy produces a sudden, irreversible additional 10% to 15% drop in production.

Half of testosterone production comes from the ovaries, and this contribution is sorely missed when it is lost. Any surgery to the fallopian tubes (tubal ligation or ectopic pregnancy) and ovaries (ovarian cystectomy or salpingo-oophorectomy) will reduce testosterone production. Weight gain increases estrogen production and produces a double whammy on testosterone levels in some women. More estrogen means more SHBG, and increased SHBG preferentially binds free testosterone over estrogen and results in reduced free testosterone. And as I'll continue to say, BHRT is all about achieving the optimal balance.

Is it any wonder that the most common patient I see in my hormone clinic is an attractive, intelligent, capable, 40-something woman, who complains that her libido has gotten up and left, like Elvis after a concert?

SEX, LOVE AND THE FEMALE LIBIDO

I recognize that the female sex drive is a complicated affair. For one thing, as pleasurable as sex is, most women say they get more enjoyment, satisfaction and fulfillment from the physical act of making love when they have an emotional connection to their partner. (Men do not always have this prerequisite as high on their list.)

So I always ask a woman to describe the quality of her relationship on a scale of 1 to 10 before I ask about her sex drive or libido. Most of the women in the 35-plus range report a good relationship and then bring up having a low libido (unless they are in a new relationship and the bloom is not yet off the rose). If the relationship score is 5 or lower, I will often suggest attention to it will yield more in terms of libido than testosterone. In other words, for most women, testosterone will not paper over the fact that they don't like their partner at that point in time. Counseling or moving on if the counseling fails is usually a better option.

Many of their relationships begin to suffer when their low sex drive does not match their partners. And here's where the whole "men are from Mars" thing comes into play: Men view sex as the physical expression of the couple's emotional bond, and can't help wonder what is wrong if their life partner doesn't return their desire for sex. All women know intuitively that men are emotionally simple creatures; this is just another example of this principle.

There is no sense arguing whether this is right or wrong, it just is what it is.

Most of the women I see are distressed about the situation, and it's usually one of the top three things they want to address. And to say a woman is happier when BHRT works and her libido is restored at or above her partner's again is an understatement. But it's important to keep something else in mind: Testosterone therapy for women is about much more than "just" sex.

THE DEEP, DARK SECRET PHARMACEUTICAL COMPANIES DON'T WANT YOU TO KNOW

Earlier, I said I don't believe in the conspiracy theories about pharmaceutical companies and medical research. And that's true. But at the same time, I think it's important to remember they are in business to make money – and there is big money being made from treating the symptoms of depression. In fact, the sale of antidepressants is the third-ranked therapy in the world – and North America has been the dominant market since 20021.

Let's start by reviewing the symptoms of androgen insufficiency:

- Flattened mood

- Decreased motivation

- Decreased sense of well being

- Persistent unexplained fatigue

- Decreased libido with a marked decrease in sexual desire or fantasy

Now, if you went to your family doctor with this list, you'd probably be told that he or she sees these same symptoms all day long. And, applying the old saying, "If all you have is a hammer, every problem looks like a nail," you would probably be described an antidepressant.

However, even if your doctor recognized androgen insufficiency, there are no pharmaceutical preparations for testosterone replacement for women at this time because, in its natural form, it can't be patented. Bioidentical testosterone is natural testosterone without the great profit point. Any pharmaceutical company in the world can make it, but this level of competition doesn't allow great profitability In process at this time are applications for transdermal testosterone patches for women. A patent could be obtained for the patch matrix release system allowing for a suitable profit margin for the company that successfully patents it. Stay tuned as much is in development, however, these patches will not address the concomitant application of estriol and in my opinion, will be inferior to compounded Biest and testosterone.

Fear not, for pharmaceutical testosterone products are being worked on with great intensity as we sit here. I do believe that, in the near future, there will be a sudden surge in pharmaceutical testosterone treatments available, and their popularity will increase. Unfortunately, we may see a repeat of the WHI if a chemically altered testosterone becomes the first to market. I suspect this won't be the case, as the WHI lessons will be well remembered. The end result of the WHI was that Wyeth ceased to be a company, as it was bought out by Pfizer Pharmaceuticals.

But this also means that antidepressants are the soup du jour of treatments for these symptoms at this time.

WHAT THAT MEANS TO YOU

The problem is, while antidepressants cover up the symptoms they do nothing to restore vitality and energy as testosterone does. And sex is not just for 24-year-olds. Many middle-aged couples report their sex lives improve as they age, especially when testosterone is used to improve the female side of the equation. Life can become simpler, and the enjoyment of sex can increase as well. After all, gone are the worries of pregnancy, the children are grown up, and the best part of grandchildren is you can love them and leave them.

Also, women's confidence tends to improve once financial security has been reached. A 2006 survey by the American Association of Retired Persons showed that adults over 40 believe sex is for every age. Sex is an important part of their lives and an important determinant of quality of life. Even women 70 and older can continue to have satisfying sex lives, and if they don't, they wish they did.

And of course, Viagra has improved many men's sex lives as they age.

It is important to mention that a high sex drive is not a prerequisite for a happy life. Many happy couples are content to let that part of life slowly fade away. Hopefully, by now, we recognize there are many ways to lead a satisfying and complete life. But this discussion is for those individuals and couples who feel their sexual health can be improved.

Even without the consideration of sexual health, I believe testosterone replacement is a critical component of a health-promotion program.

TESTOSTERONE – IT'S NOT JUST FOR SEX ANY MORE

Something important to remember is that testosterone has many targets other than the brain center for libido. Heart, bone, muscles, the entire brain, nipples, clitoris, vagina and a host of other tissues all have testosterone receptors for a reason.

For example, did you know that without enough testosterone in your system, your:

- Arteries are more likely to harden

- Blood pressure can go out of control (and be more difficult to manage)

- Blood flow to your heart decreases and your heart muscle gets weaker

But that's not all.

Some benefits of regaining your optimal levels of testosterone:

- Enjoy higher, longer-lasting energy levels

- Add more lean muscle mass to increase your metabolism and help you lose weight

- Lose that tummy bulge

- Skin looks and feels younger

- Regain your zest and lust for life

- Feel happier naturally without expensive pills or risky side effects

I prescribe transdermal testosterone because it doesn't increase SHBG and allows adequate delivery to the body. Now let's go into where testosterone goes in the body and what it does when it gets there.

YOUR BRAIN ON TESTOSTERONE

Testosterone has powerful, beneficial effects in the brain. Animal studies have shown an increase in brain cell growth and increased development of connections with the use of testosterone. A significant number of animal studies show improved cognitive abilities thanks to testosterone, and we know it also has a role in the improvement and preservation of self-confidence and assertiveness. This appears to be a result of an increase in dopamine, one of the brain's primary neurotransmitters. These are the same neurotransmitters targeted by many of the antidepressant medications. Remember how much androgen insufficiency looks like depression?

BREAST HEALTH

Chapter 11 included more detailed information on the effects of testosterone on the breasts. But it's important to point out that recent editorials have suggested that the evidence is sufficient to recommend the addition of testosterone to HRT. I believe the evidence is strong and robust. There really should be no debate.

It's also important to mention that some recent studies show that women should not take SSRI antidepressants if they have had breast cancer and are receiving tamoxifen therapy to cut down the risk of recurrence. SSRIs are selective serotonin reuptake inhibitors and include fluoxetine (Prozac), paroxetine (Paxil) and sertraline (Zoloft).

Because tamoxifen can often cause severe hot flushes, SSRIs are routinely prescribed to help with them and with depression. New evidence shows that some of these drugs are potent inhibitors of the cytochrome P450 2D6 enzyme, which converts tamoxifen to its active metabolite, endoxifen. By inhibiting the enzyme, these drugs reduce the blood levels of the active metabolite, which reduces the ability of tamoxifen to protect against breast cancer recurrence.

One such study, conducted in collaboration with researchers from Indiana University, used Medco's 11 million-member database to identify 945 women older than 50 and who were at least 70% compliant with tamoxifen therapy for two years or more. The researchers identified an additional 353 such women who were also taking an SSRI (most commonly paroxetine or fluoxetine); the median overlap during which they were taking both drugs was 255 days. The study showed "significant difference" in the risk of breast cancer recurrence between women who were taking SSRIs and those who were not – 16% v. 7% respectively.

Other studies show that the SSRIs that have only a weak inhibitory effect on the enzyme had only an 8.8% risk for breast cancer recurrence, not significantly different from the 7.5% seen in women who did not take these drugs. Weak inhibitors of the enzyme include citalopram (Celexa), escitalopram (Lexapro) and fluvoxamine (Luvox).

However, since transdermal testosterone provides therapeutic effect and does not interfere with the 2D6 enzyme, antidepressants may not be necessary at all – this is something to discuss with your doctor.

CARDIOVASCULAR HEALTH

In Chapter 10, we reviewed hormone data as it relates to heart health. We know that removal of the ovaries at time of hysterectomy decreases testosterone production significantly – and corresponds to a significant increase in heart disease in these women.

The evidence is strong enough that many of us gynecologists do not routinely remove ovaries in women under the age of 60 for the prevention of ovarian cancer; the procedure reduces the risk but does not eliminate it. In most cases, the benefit of removal is far outweighed by the increased rates of heart disease and stroke seen in these women. Remember, statistically speaking, after menopause, cardiovascular disease is what will likely disable or kill you.

OSTEOPOROSIS

There is no debate in the literature for testosterone and bone density. Osteoblasts, or bone cells, have testosterone receptors. Higher levels of testosterone increase osteoblast activity – and lead to increased bone formation.

At this time, testosterone's effect appears to be more pronounced than any other product sold for prevention and treatment of osteoporosis (thin, weak bones that are prone to fracture). The effects of testosterone and estrogen are complimentary for bone health. The combination of the two hormones is better at maintaining and building bone density than either alone.

MUSCLE MASS

Whenever I mention muscle mass, I can see alarmed women thinking they do not want to look like Arnold Schwarzenegger during his body-building days. Rest assured, this is not what we are talking about.

One of the most common conditions associated with aging is sarcopenia, the medical label for loss of muscle mass. It has some rather severe consequences. For one thing, our muscle mass determines our metabolic rate – and it is improved with weight training and BHRT.

A higher metabolic rate allows us to burn more calories, rather than store them (which means you stay leaner, stronger, and can maintain a healthy weight even as you get older). It also reduces your chances of having significant levels of inflammatory compounds or excess estrogen from your fat tissues – which is not good as you age.

I think this is one of the more exciting aspects of BHRT, and hope it gets much more attention in the future. Sarcopenia leads to weakness and weakness leads to falls. Falls create fractures and fractures lead to disability, nursing-home care and death. I believe BHRT with testosterone has a huge role to play in this area as preventative medicine.

If technologic advances lead to significant life extension, as many experts in the area believe, we will need to actively look for ways to maintain and improve our quality of life as well – or what's the point of living longer?

THE NUTS AND BOLTS OF TESTOSTERONE THERAPY

I prescribe testosterone only as a cream – either on its own or with Biest. I have found application of the cream to the vulva provides the most efficient and predictable absorption. Other areas of the skin were my starting point, but the shift to vulvar application showed better and more predictable results, even with lower doses. I've found a starting dose of 1-2 mg per day is a good beginning.

Eight weeks after the initiation or modification of therapy, I run a 12-hour free-testosterone-level blood test. I aim for a level of 10 picamoles/liter (3.1 pg/decalitre) and adjust it according to the patient's symptoms. To do the test, I ask women to apply the testosterone cream at bedtime for three days before. Blood is drawn the next morning to sample the testosterone level roughly 10-12 hours after application.

This allows an accurate estimate of testosterone supplementation that can be used to guide therapy. The levels we see with this test line up well with a symptom chart that is used in all patients. The symptom chart is essential for the proper BHRT treatment because we are treating people, NOT lab results. Symptoms are interpreted in light of blood levels to give us the whole picture.

Testosterone can be compounded with Biest in the post-menopausal women or used on its own for estrogen-dominant women.

The vulva has no hair, so there is no issue with coarsening and darkening of body hair. I have had very few reports of vaginal discharge or irritation. If such problems crop up, switch application every other day to another area, such as the pubis or legs, where hair darkening is not as much of a problem.

The vast majority of women report significant improvement in energy, mental sharpness, mood and libido after using testosterone for six to eight weeks.

MEASURING TESTOSTERONE

There are several methods of reporting testosterone results, and each with pros and cons.

Total testosterone: This includes free and bound testosterone (albumin and SHBG). This test is not very accurate for women and I do not recommend this method. It is a cheap test, but hormone measurement is like much of life: You get what you pay for.

Bioavailable testosterone: This test is the same as above, but includes a calculation to remove the portion bound to albumin and SHBG. The methodology is much the same as total testosterone, which means accuracy is a concern.

Salivary testosterone: This is a great test if you're not already on treatment for the initial visit. It provides baseline information regarding estrogen, progesterone, cortisol and DHEA. However, I believe the science for measurement when a woman is already on testosterone treatment is poor and therefore I cannot recommend it. Many practitioners use this test, and it is the method of monitoring BHRT suggested by the American Academy of Anti-Aging. I believe the cost places serious limits on its use in Canada, and I do not use this method to monitor my patients on treatment with testosterone. Remember, in Canada blood tests for hormone levels are free while saliva tests are not free

Free testosterone: This is my choice for monitoring women on testosterone treatment. It has great accuracy down to the pmol/liter values that need to be measured. The test must be done by a complicated methodology called equilibrium dialysis. I am fortunate to work in a health region that uses this test for free testosterone. The test is free for my patients, as I work in Canada, and it satisfies my need to measure all the treatments I prescribe for a patient.

ALTERNATIVE TESTOSTERONE TREATMENT OPTIONS

Oral: Not effective and full of potential problems. This route of testosterone administration is not recommended.

Patch: One is supposed to be in the later stages of development. However, when it becomes available I predict two immediate consequences: First, we will be inundated with messages about the epidemic of androgen insufficiency in women. (And until it's available, why spend money on a problem you don't have a fix for?) And second, it will be very expensive. (Remember sex is a luxury and luxuries are not cheap.)

Pellets: These are a good option for those with an experienced practitioner and a compounding pharmacy that can make them at a reasonable cost. Unfortunately, those two conditions do not exist in my area. However, if they're available where you are, the pellets can have estrogen, progesterone and testosterone placed in them. They are inserted under the skin and will work for four to six months. They are convenient and closely mimic the way nature delivers hormones. The biggest problem is that you have no "days off" your treatment. Once they've been inserted, you receive the hormones for the life of the pellet.

REAL WOMEN, REAL STORIES

C. H.

Shortly after I had turned 50, I started menopause. With my mother passing away from breast and ovarian cancer as well as an aunt on my dad's side dying at a young age of breast cancer, HRT was out of the question. I tried to do it on my own, drug free. I went four years of struggling with hot flashes, insomnia and mood swings, as well as depression. My only solution, I thought, was sleeping pills to help sleep and antidepressants for the other problems. I did resort to sleeping pills on occasion, after going all week with hardly any sleep, but I didn't want to go on anti-depressants. I had read and heard of bioidentical hormone replacement. After meeting Dr. Brown and telling him how miserable I was feeling and that I could not take HRT, he started me on the bioidentical, which is more natural. It took three months, but I finally started to feel good. He watches my estrogen levels because I'm at such a high risk for breast and ovarian cancer. My youngest sister has since had breast cancer and a mastectomy, as well.

With his help, I have to say what a difference a year makes. It has been that long now since I first met with Dr. Brown and I am feeling good. I have not taken sleeping pills since. Thanks for giving me my life back.

In summary

- Testosterone production falls in women from the age of 25 to menopause.

- Each pregnancy causes a 10% to 15% nonreversible decline in testosterone production.

- Oral estrogen, in the form of the birth control pill or with HRT, reduces free testosterone.

- Low free testosterone results in the symptoms of androgen insufficiency.

- Sex can be an important part of life into the 70s and 80s.

- Testosterone treatment improves libido, energy, and the zest for life that many lose as they age.

- Testosterone has health benefits for the brain, muscles, bones and heart.

- Testosterone therapy is simple and safe.

- It's not all about sex!

CHAPTER 15

TESTOSTERONE THERAPY IN MEN

This has been one of the strangest chapters to write. After all, I am a gynecologist, so what would I know about treating men with BHRT?

Actually, it all has to do with the nature of women. Women have an innate desire to share. So when a woman encounters a treatment or measure that improves her quality of life, she naturally shares it with friends and family. This has been true with bioidentical hormones.

As my patients begin to see improvements in their symptoms, one can almost see the light bulb go on. Their first instinct is to share this new approach with girlfriends, sisters and mothers. And the next logical connection is, of course, their spouses or partners. In fact, as the woman's energy and libido improves, it often becomes necessary for her partner to also seek treatment to rebalance the libido equation.

And that's how it has gone with my bioidentical hormone practice – male partners and spouses began to regularly turn up looking for the same kinds of treatments that they have watched dramatically improve their partner's quality of life.

As you can imagine, this originally made me feel a bit uncomfortable and out of my element! Of course, by the time I started getting more and more male patients, I'd already tried the testosterone treatment myself and had become a believer after seeing what a difference it made in my own well being.

This is actually very typical for practitioners in the field. You learn a bit, try it out on yourself first, and then move on to family and friends. But, it had been 20 years since I had treated men – back in my early family practice days. Talk about unfamiliar territory! My studies of BHRT had covered male treatment in depth, but I have to admit I still felt a little uneasy. What did I know any more about prostate problems and testosterone therapy?

However, as is usually the case when a problem presents itself, there was a solution nearby, just waiting to be discovered. It came in my discovery of a new book about testosterone therapy in men. I had already read several others, and while they were informative, I never felt completely ready to jump into the field.

Testosterone For Life: Recharge Your Vitality, Sex Drive, Muscle Mass, and Overall Health, by Dr. Abraham Morgentaler was like a breath of fresh air. The best teachers understand their subject so well that they're able to distill it down into easily understood concepts. Dr. Morgentaler was able to do this for me on this subject. I will try to do the same for you.

We are talking about male menopause, or andropause. Just as women's hormones decline from age 25 on, so too does testosterone production in men, though they do not experience the hormone swings that women do during menopause.

For women, the change is dramatic and demands recognition. For men, the subtle and gradual changes can be easily missed and are often put down to just getting older. However, as our life expectancy continues to increase, the concept of hormonal imbalances becomes more important.

While it's true that the drop in hormone production is natural, it creates disease and disability. And when you begin to look at the big picture, the overall loss of productivity and lowered quality of life is staggering, all the more so because there are simple and inexpensive methods to correct and rebalance the hormones.

So, if there is a simple fix, why is this area of treatment for men being overlooked? Several factors act together, in this regard.

The first, of course, is a lack of recognition that there is even a problem. The second has to do with the male psyche and the relationship of testosterone to sex and self-esteem. And the third obstacle is the association of testosterone therapy and prostate cancer and heart disease.

ANDROGEN DEFICIENCY

Androgen deficiency is the relative or absolute deficiency of testosterone or its metabolites according to the needs of an individual at a specific time in his life – in this case, once a man reaches middle age.

Next, it's important to understand that as we age, there are certain resistance factors in the body to the action of testosterone. These factors actively antagonize the actions of testosterone at the cellular level. They include:

- Increased sex-hormone binding globulin (this hormone-transport protein doubles in levels from age 20 to 60 and results in significant reductions in free testosterone)

- Stress and rising cortisol levels

- Obesity and increased estrogen production

- Increased exposure to environmental xenoestrogens

- Reduced androgen receptor function

Also, as men age, testosterone production gradually falls and eventually intersects with rising resistance, and symptoms develop. The rest of this chapter will address the treatment to reduce the subtle symptoms.

The figure below summarizes these concepts quite clearly, and is based on the concept of active aging put forward by the World Health Organization. The heart of the issue is to decrease the rate of decline in functional capacity. Any measures to flatten the decline will increase the amount of time the individual will maintain independence in activities of daily living. This is completely in line with the desires of most people. They do not want to hear that aging associated with infirmity and reduced quality of life. The present day medical model pays lip service to these concepts but at times preservation of the status quo seems to be the priority. In my opinion, the present day model serves physicians and drug companies more than the people they are meant to serve.

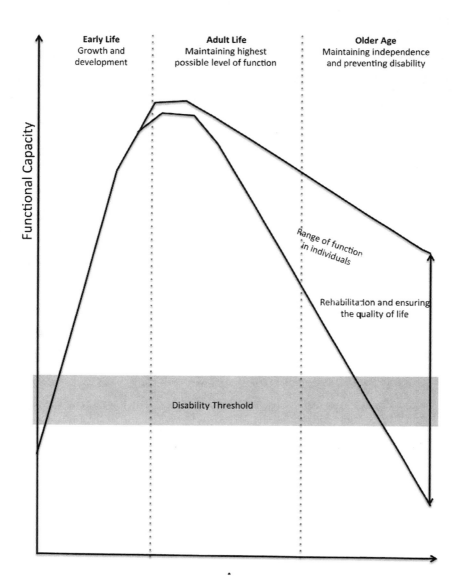

Fig. 15-1: Functional capacity

This concept is at the core of bioidentical hormone therapy and is simply stated as "therapies and interventions aimed at supporting optimal function in early life, middle age and old age."

It is hard to argue with this concept, yet much of modern medicine does just that. The figure compares mental and physical function throughout life to that of the flight of a glider. Within the broad range of normal testosterone production, many factors compete to change the glide path trajectory.

The rate of descent, which at this time seems inevitable, but in fact may not be, is influenced by many factors. Thermal up-currents include success at work and love, recreation and relaxation. The opposing factors include stress, mental or physical inactivity, and illness. All of these factors combine to give each individual his own flight path. This is all superimposed on the 50% decline of free testosterone from age 25 to 75[1].

Great steps were taken toward clinical recognition of andropause as recently as 1998. The First World Congress on the Aging Male brought together experts from around the world. Consensus was reached and further World Congress events have given us a definition and treatment recommendations. The most important symptoms of testosterone deficiency in men over 50 are, in decreasing order of importance:

- Loss of libido

- Erectile dysfunction

- Depression

- Reduced cognitive function

- Osteoporosis

- Reduced muscle mass

These symptoms are correlated with testosterone levels to make the diagnosis.

Much progress has been made in the recognition of this area. Most notably, articles in major medical journals have greatly increased physician awareness[2]. We now recognize that androgen deficiency is a multi-factorial problem that is best considered with a look at all the levels influencing testosterone production and function.

AGING

The brain is the biggest sex organ. As we age, changes in cognitive function, psychological issues and reduced penile sensitivity all conspire against us. Stress has been consistently shown to negatively influence testosterone production. However, stressful situations that result in a rise in status lead to increased production of testosterone and vice versa. Also, chronic low-grade stress, such as financial issues, relationship issues, and the loss of friends and relatives, acts to decrease production.

DRUGS

All antidepressants, anxiolytic, antiepileptic and antipsychotic drugs reduce testosterone production. Also, blood-pressure-lowering agents and diuretics adversely influence testosterone secretion.

HYPOTHALAMUS AND PITUITARY

Numerous changes result in the loss of rhythmicity of gonadotropin secretion. The brain produces gonadotropins to direct the testicles to produce testosterone. As men age, the secretion is altered, negatively affecting testosterone production. Also, increased sensitivity to negative feedback of the sex hormones conspires to reduce testosterone production.

ALCOHOL

Many people are surprised to find that mild-to-moderate, long-term levels of alcohol intake actually improve overall testosterone production. Alcohol over time creates a change in the liver metabolism that increases the conversion of androstenedione to testosterone. But in contrast, excess alcohol intake – short- or long-term – has been shown to reduce testosterone production.

The adverse effect of heavy alcohol intake is likely mediated by increased oxidative stress and its metabolic consequences, as well as the increased oxidative damage to brain and testicular tissue. Increased estrogen production is also seen with excess, chronic alcohol intake. As we have seen before, estrogen is a direct antagonist to testosterone and its natural effects. Estrogen antagonizes the actions of testosterone in men just as effectively as what we have seen previously in women. And xenoestrogens from the environment directly reduce testosterone production.

TESTES

Vasectomy seems to have a direct but delayed negative effect on testosterone production by the testicles.

These effects can be seen as much as 10-20 years after the operation and may be – at least in part – mediated by auto-antibodies such as anti-sperm antibodies.

This is still an area of great controversy, and the negative effect is not great. Vascular disease with reduction of blood supply to the testes as a result of arterial narrowing and blockage is another negative factor. These processes are particularly prominent in diabetic and hypertensive men.

MAKING THE DIAGNOSIS

So how, then, do we diagnose androgen deficiency in men? The diagnosis is based on a platform with two main planks. The first is a questionnaire that determines whether there are significant symptoms to support the diagnosis. The second is blood testing.

Of the many questionnaires available, I favor Androgen Deficiency in Aging Males, developed by Morley[3]. It is limited as a tool for research into comparison of different treatment options. But, since I'm not involved in this type of research, its simplicity wins the day.

Do You Have Low Testosterone?

ADAM, Androgen Deficiency in Aging Men

1.DO you have a decrease in libido (sex drive)?	Yes	No
2.Do you have a lack of energy?	Yes	No
3.Do you have a decrease in strength and/or endurance?	Yes	No
4.Have you lost height?	Yes	No
5.Have you noticed a decreased enjoyment of life?	Yes	No
6.Are you sad and/or grumpy?	Yes	No
7.Are your erections less strong?	Yes	No
8. During sexual intercourse, has it been more difficult to maintain your erection to completion of intercourse?	Yes	No
9. Are you falling asleep after dinner?	Yes	No
10.Has there been a recent deterioration in your work performance?	Yes	No

If you answered yes to questions 1 or 7, or at least three of the other questions you may have low testosterone levels. Fortunately there is something your doctor can do to help. Be sure to discuss the results of this quiz with your doctor.

Table 15-1: Androgen deficiency

My experience with this format has been completely positive. Men are not honest with direct questions in these matters. They will NEVER tell you the "state of the union," whether it is a male or female practitioner asking the questions. Yet men have no trouble answering a questionnaire such as this in a straightforward fashion.

If the symptoms of androgen deficiency exist, the next step is the laboratory evaluation. Total, bioavailable and free testosterone can all be measured, and each has its pros and cons. The weight of many studies and lines of evidence favor free testosterone, and that is the measure I use. Interested readers are directed toward an excellent analysis of this area by Carruthers[4]. Significant symptoms, along with a free testosterone in the lower one-third of the reference range, clinch the diagnosis and allow us to consider therapy. This illustrates one of the central tenets of treatment with bioidentical hormones. The normal range for most hormones is quite wide, as they are established using the bell curve that groups 95% of results as "normal." We need to move on to the concept of "optimal" range where we can show ideal function in tissues responsive to a particular hormone. Some men may have optimal function in the lower 1/3 of the normal range, while others may not function in an optimal fashion unless they are in the upper 1/3 of the normal range. Tests results need to be interpreted in light of a patient's symptoms and function. Practicing medicine on the basis of antiquated lab ranges is just not good enough for this millennium!

One concept that will attract a lot of attention in the future is that of an "individual reference" range for each man. Men have a wide distribution of testosterone levels from about age 25. Symptoms of androgen insufficiency may depend on the reduction in testosterone an individual experiences in life, referenced back to his optimal level at 20-25.

High T-level men may develop symptoms with testosterone levels at the 50th percentile. Conversely, low T- level men may not be symptomatic even in the lower fifth of the reference range, if this level doesn't reflect a significant drop from levels earlier in life. This is why the symptoms questionnaire is central to the diagnosis. It allows us to reference back to what is normal to that particular man in the absence of the ability to measure his testosterone levels in his mid-20s. It's interesting to note that this concept likely applies to women as well. There are high- and low-estrogen, -progesterone and -testosterone women. Treatment based on blood levels allows us to be misled, since it doesn't reference treatment back to the individual. My children have had their levels checked in early adulthood for this very reason.

Any male with symptoms of androgen deficiency deserves a proper trial of androgen treatment. It is a clinical, not a laboratory, diagnosis!

Male self-esteem is perhaps more complicated than that of women, and any discussion of sex drive with men runs right into a wall. Unfortunately, society and men themselves equate maleness with sex. Men equate strength of erection with maleness, and this forms a central part of their view of self. Ask a man directly if he has problems with erections and the answer is always NO. Then glance at his questionnaire and he will have answered YES.

I no longer ask the question, as I hate to waste the patient's and my own time. Why go through the charade? Just look at the questionnaire and free-testosterone levels and draw your conclusion. I will validate the answers with the patient in a nondirect fashion and explain what we are looking for from the treatment. Men don't want to talk about the problem; they want to talk about the solution.

The next obstacle to the recognition of the male andropause is the association of testosterone with heart disease and prostate cancer. This stems from the observation that men have more heart disease than women and they can suffer from prostate cancer. Dr. Morgentaler's book is an excellent resource to dispel these myths of the association.

Suffice it to say, the evidence is overwhelming: Testosterone therapy reduces the incidence of heart disease and prostate cancer. Prostate cancer is the manifestation of LOW testosterone levels relative to estrogen over a period of years. It is certainly more complicated than this simple summary. Indeed, conversion of testosterone to the very powerful dihydrotestosterone (DHT) may be an important factor in the genesis of prostate cancer. Much more is to be written in this area over the next few years.

TESTOSTERONE TREATMENT

One of the guiding principles of medicine is that of first, do no harm. To proceed safely with androgen treatment, an evaluation of symptoms, history and laboratory results are combined with physical exam. Safe treatment also involves careful monitoring of the effects of treatment. Many studies have looked at the safety of testosterone therapy and have uniformly shown it to be one of the safest forms of treatment.

Carruthers' book[4] has an excellent section for those interested in the details. The major goal of therapy was stated by the Workshop Conference on Androgen Therapy[5]. The consensus view was that therapy should replace testosterone levels at as close to physiologic concentrations as possible.

Here is a summary of the International Society for the Study of the Aging Male(ISSAM) in a recent article on treatment guidelines:

Serum samples for bioavailable or free testosterone drawn from 8-11 a.m. are the recommended choice. Testosterone values below the accepted value of normal should be repeated with LH, prolactin and FSH added.

A clear indication – supported with a clinical picture and bio-chemical values – should exist prior to initiation of androgen therapy. Age is not a limiting factor in the consideration of ART (androgen replacement therapy). Currently available preparations of testosterone (with the exception of alkylated ones) are safe and effective. The treating physician should have an adequate understanding of the advantages and drawbacks of each preparation.

Liver function tests are advisable before, quarterly during the first year, and on a yearly basis during treatment. A fasting lipid profile prior to start of therapy, and yearly while on treatment, should also be done. Digital rectal exam (DRE) and determination of prostate-specific antigen (PSA) are mandatory in men older than 40 prior to therapy, quarterly in the first year, and yearly while on treatment. Tran-srectal ultrasound-guided biopsies of the prostate are indicated only if the DRE or PSA are abnormal.

Urologic consultation should be arranged if there is:

- An increase in PSA of more than 1.5 ng/ml/year, verified on repeat testing

- An average annual increase of more than .75 ng/ml over a minimum of two years

- A PSA of more than 4.0 ng/ml

CONTRAINDICATIONS OF ANDROGEN THERAPY

Androgen administration is absolutely contraindicated in men suspected of prostate or breast cancer or men with severe bladder neck obstruction due to a benign, enlarged prostate. Moderate obstruction represents a partial contraindication. The following chart is a useful predictive guide to the possibility of prostate enlargement. If prostatic enlargement is present, testosterone therapy may worsen the symptoms. Discontinuation of the testosterone will allow the problem to resolve and he should be promptly referred to his family doctor.

International Prostate Symptom Score (IPSS)

Please answer the following questions about your urinary symptoms
Write your score for each question at the end of each row..

Over the past month how often have you..	Not at all	Less than 1 time in . 5	Less than half the time	About Half the time	More than half the time	Almost always	Your score
1. Has a sensation of not emptying your bladder completely after you finish urinating?	0	1	2	3	4	5	
2. Had to urinate again less than to hours after you finished urinating?	0	1	2	3	4	5	
3. Stopped and started again several times?	0	1	2	3	4	5	
4.Found it difficult to postpone urination?	0	1	2	3	4	5	
5. Had a weak urinary stream?	0	1	2	3	4	5	
6. Had to push or strain to begin urination?	0	1	2	3	4	5	
And finally...	None	once	twice	3 times	4 times	5 or more times	
7. Over the past month, how many times did you most typically get up to urinate from the time you went to bed at night until the time you got up in the morning?	0	1	2	3	4	5	
Add up your total score and write it in the box.							

The result from this questionnaire will help your doctor to assess if you have an enlarged prostate. This is a common and benign condition that often occurs in older men. In general, a score of.

-0-7 indicates mild symptoms
-8-19 indicates moderate symptoms
-20-35 indicates severe symptoms
See your doctor to discuss the results if your score indicates moderate or severe symptoms.

Table 15-2: IPSS scores

The development of negative behavioral patterns, including increased anger or emotional liability, during treatment calls for dose modification or discontinuation of treatment. This is almost never seen in my experience.

Increased hemoglobin occasionally develops on treatment. Periodic hematologic monitoring is needed and dose adjustments may be required.

Safety data for ART in men with sleep apnea is insufficient. Good clinical judgment and caution should be employed in this situation. Monitoring during ART is a shared responsibility; the physician must emphasize to the patient the need for periodic evaluations and the patient must comply.

TESTOSTERONE PREPARATIONS

Injections: Free testosterone is not useful as an injectable agent, as its half-life is about 10 minutes. The addition of fatty-acid side chains produced compounds with a longer half-life and include:

- Testosterone propionate

- Testosterone cypionate

- Testosterone enanthate

Testosterone enanthate is the injectable form most fully researched and has tremendous worldwide clinical evidence on safety. The most common dose is 250 mg given every two weeks. Most patients will be happy with their symptom response.

The chart below demonstrates the different blood levels seen with the various treatment intervals.

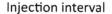

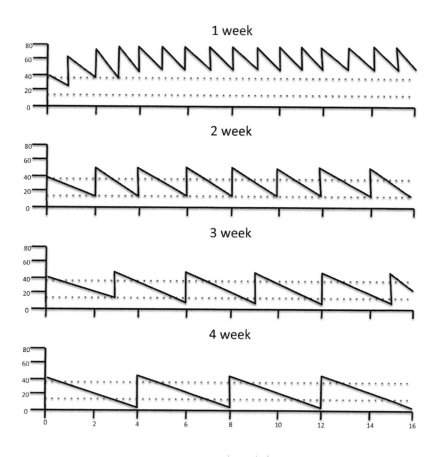

Fig. 15-2: Testosterone blood levels

Oral preparations: Pure testosterone taken orally is well absorbed, but is broken down in the liver. Methyl-testosterone was developed in the 1970s, but was discovered to be toxic to the liver and heart.

Further research led to the development of testosterone undecanoate (Andriol), which is a pill form of testosterone. It appears to be most useful in the aging man for whom testosterone levels just need to be topped up. A dose of 80-200 mg per day is effective and safe for treating most andropausal men. A 40 mg capsule of Andriol is equivalent to 25 mg of testosterone.

It is important that it be taken with food, preferably with some fat to improve absorption. If it's taken on an empty stomach, almost no absorption occurs. It is recommended that the largest dose (2/3) be taken with breakfast and the remainder at lunch. Taking Andriol with the evening meal can result in insomnia. Start with 80 mg at breakfast and 40 mg with lunch. The dosage is titrated up to a maximum of 120 mg twice per day, especially in overweight patients. Capsules should be stored at room temperature for optimal absorption.

In studies of the effects of treatment with Andriol a significant rise in DHT was seen, with no rise in estradiol. Also, we see a consistent fall in SHBG with this preparation. These two effects result in a proportionally greater rise in free testosterone than with other preparations, which greatly enhances its therapeutic effect. The patient should be reassessed at three months with a blood sample at least three hours after the morning dose. There is a considerable body of safety evidence for this product.

Testosterone implants: Pellet implants were one of the first forms of testosterone therapy. They have a long history and documented safety. Doses need to increase with age due to the increase in SHBG. Young men with testicular failure respond well to 600-750 (8-10 pellets) mg every four-six months, while older men may need 750-1,200 (10-16 pellets) mg every three to six months for an optimal response.

The pellets are inserted into a small incision on the upper, outer quadrant of the buttocks. Symptomatic improvement is seen within

10-14 days, and the pellets are reinserted in three to-six months when symptoms start to reappear. Continuation rates of 90% are seen with this approach, reflecting the convenience and effectiveness of pellets. This continuation rate is despite soreness at the site of injection for 7-10 days.

Transdermal cream: Testosterone cream compounded by a pharmacy is an effective method for about 80% of men. Absorption through the thick stratum corneum of the skin in men is a problem, and requires significant doses of 20-200 mg per day to achieve adequate blood levels. These doses are similar to those seen with Andriol, and reflect the relative inefficiency of this delivery route. With both the oral and transdermal routes, we can expect wastage of 50%-95% of the manufactured dose.

Cream application to the inner forearm and flank region is recommended in the morning to minimize transfer to the female partner. Changes in timing of sex may require a change of application timing.

An Australian company, Lawley Pharmaceuticals, produces a range of testosterone creams for men. Andromen with 20 mg/g and Andromen Forte with 50 mg/g are available in North America. These can circumvent the issues of quality control that are cited by opponents of compounding pharmacies. I have had no issues with compounding pharmacy quality control, and feel this has been well-monitored by blood-level testing.

Scrotal patches (Testoderm): A patch can improve the absorption of testosterone. Studies showed 40 times the absorption using the scrotum as compared to the chest. Scrotal skin is thinner and has a better-developed blood supply that is advantageous for absorption.

This is quite analogous to use of the vulva for testosterone application in women.

Due to high levels of 5-alpha reductase activity in scrotal skin, DHT levels increase two-three times with this product. There appears to be no adverse consequence.

Skin gels: These are the latest development in testosterone therapy. Alcoholic gels rapidly dry and leave the testosterone on the skin to be absorbed more slowly. Poor absorption is still an issue, however, with only 9%-14% absorption seen. Cost is also another factor, as compared with their compounded counterparts. Slow absorption also increases the chances of transfer to a female partner and resultant over-dosage of testosterone in the woman.

PROSTATE SAFETY

This has long been a deterrent to testosterone therapy in the minds of physicians. However, the historical linkage of testosterone with prostate cancer is factually untrue. Dr. Morgentaler's book *Testosterone for Life: Recharge Your Vitality, Sex Drive, Muscle Mass, and Overall Health*, looks deeply into this area to dispel the myths. By following the treatment guidelines listed above, the risk is minimal to nonexistent.

In a review article by Frick[6] in 1998, all short-term studies of ART showed no change in PSA, prostate size or urine flow rate. A 2003 review by Kaufman[7] reviewed data from eight prospective studies and found: "While a definitive conclusion regarding the long-term safety of androgen supplementation in aging men is not possible, available data support the safety of such treatment in the short term. No evidence of increased risk for clinical prostate cancer or symptomatic BPH has been found in trials lasting up to three years."

CARDIOVASCULAR SAFETY

As long as methyl-testosterone is avoided, all the evidence points to heart safety. Indeed, correctly administered ART appears to promote cardiovascular health. Testosterone appears to have an anti-atherogenic effect on the coronary arteries. Testosterone also appears to reduce large artery stiffness, which in turn reduces blood pressure, a known causative factor in heart disease.

A large epidemiologic study by English[8] showed that men with coronary heart disease have significantly reduced levels of androgens. It also showed that low-dose testosterone-patch treatment improved exercise-induced heart ischemia in men with stable angina [9].

On balance, testosterone appears to be heart-healthy and may find a role in the future for treatment of existing heart disease in men.

Important Points

1. The andropause is real and is the result of gradually declining testosterone levels from age 25.

2. Declining testosterone levels decrease quality of life and increase the chances of heart disease and prostate cancer.

3. Other changes in a man's physiology as he ages conspire to further reduce free or bioavailable testosterone.

4. Androgen insufficiency in the male is a defined disorder and is characterized by:

   • Loss of libido

   • Erectile dysfunction

   • Depression

   • Decreased cognitive function

   • Osteoporosis

   • Decreased muscle mass

5. Testosterone replacement is to be considered if symptoms and corroborating blood work support the diagnosis.

6. Symptoms are the most important factor in determining the need for treatment.

7. Injections, pellets, tablets, cream and patches are all acceptable methods of androgen replacement therapy (ART). Each modality has pros and cons and should be chosen for the individual.

8. Digital rectal exam and PSA measurements should be done before initiation of treatment, and at regular intervals on treatment.

9. Abnormalities in either should necessitate urologic consultation.

10. ART appears to be safe with respect to prostate cancer. New evidence suggests that prostate cancer rates increase in the setting of LOW testosterone.

11. ART appears to be cardio-protective.

12. ART can dramatically increase quality of life and should be considered in all symptomatic, aging men.

1 J Clin Endocrinol Metab 1971; 33 ; 759-67 A Vermeulen et al. / 2 Br Med J 2000; 320; 858-61 D Gould et al. / 3 Med Clin North Am 1999; 83; 1279-89 JE Morley et al. / 4 Androgen Deficiency in the Adult Male 2004 M Carruthers pg 105-30 / 5 Guidelines for the Use of Androgens 1992 WHO Geneva E Nieschlag et al. / 6 Testosterone: Action, Deficiency, Substitution 1998; 259-91 J Frick et al. / 7 Aging Male 2003; 6; 166-74 JM Kaufman / 8 Eur Heart J 2000; 21; 890-4 KM English et al. 9.Circulation 2000; 102; 1906-11 KM English et al.

CHAPTER 16

THE COMPOUNDING PHARMACY AND YOU

One of the core concepts of BHRT comes down to a team of three: You, the patient; your doctor, the BHRT practitioner; and finally, the compounding pharmacy – which is critical to the success of your BHRT.

If you're new to BHRT, you may be wondering where to find a compounding pharmacy – and chances are, you may not have realized such a thing even existed. Most of us are familiar with the Walgreens, Shoppers Drug and Costco varieties of drugstores. In days gone by, though, all local drug stores started as compounding pharmacies, and along the way, as technologies changed and improved, they morphed into the familiar stores listed above. This happened along with the change in drug manufacturing and development of the pharmaceutical industry.

However, some druggists did not stray far from their roots of preparing individualized medications for the needs of a specific patient. The ones who persisted and are still around represent our present-day compounding pharmacies. While they sell regular pharmaceuticals, their specialty lies in their creativity.

You know from reading this book that BHRT is not the one-size-fits-all approach that has become so common in the pharmaceutical approach. If you're like a lot of my patients, that actually comes as a relief – because chances are you haven't had a lot of success with the cookie-cutter treatments that you've received up to this point. Knowing that your health practitioner is going to create a customized treatment plan for you, based on your symptoms, your test results, and how well you react to the treatment over time, can bring you a lot of peace of mind.

Many BHRT prescriptions are unique and designed solely for a particular patient in terms of dose, application method, or vehicle used to deliver the therapeutic agent. This is why most BHRT practitioners develop a close working relationship with one or two compounding pharmacies.

First, the prescription must spell out what main compound is to be used (for example, Biest or Triest) and then what hormone or other substances should be added (such as testosterone, estrogen) along with the desired percentage in the formulation (80/20 or 50/50), and finally the vehicle to be used (HRT versus PLO cream).

Then the application or use instructions are added.

ARE BHRT PRODUCTS USED BY THE COMPOUNDING PHARMACY SAFE?

All of the hormones used in BHRT are pharmaceutical products produced by major drug companies. Some of these companies have chosen to specialize in this area rather than in patent or generic drugs.

Pharmaceutical companies that make hormones for the bioidentical hormone industry are held to the same high standard of drug production as traditional pharmaceutical companies. These standards include guarantee of content and potency, as well as freedom from contamination. In fact, you might be surprised to learn that some of the major pharmaceutical companies have bioidentical hormone divisions. On the surface, that would seem to be in competition with the traditional pharmaceutical divisions, don't you think?

Compounding pharmacies generally buy the hormones from associations such as the PCCA, or Professional Compounding Centers of America. This ensures the quality of the hormones going into the BHRT prescription.

HOW COMPOUNDING PHARMACIES CREATE YOUR TREATMENT

Upon getting your prescription, the compounding pharmacist has to mix the hormones into a base he or she believes is appropriate for the job. The pharmacist pays meticulous attention to detail, to create the product as spelled out in the prescription.

You may be interested to know that the flow of information between the practitioner and pharmacist is not a one-way street. For example, much of the knowledge I have gathered over the last few years is a result of interactions with the compounding pharmacies I use. In my opinion, it's better for the patient when a practitioner sticks to one or two pharmacists, because of the relationship between the two.

COMPOUNDING PHARMACIES SUBJECT TO CONTROVERSY

Unluckily, as the popularity of BHRT has continued to grow, the compounding pharmacist has become thrust into the center of controversy.

One of the strengths of the modern pharmaceutical model is the quality control of the manufacturing process. Once a drug is produced and delivered to a regular pharmacy, the only errors possible are the wrong number of pills, or dispensing of the wrong drug.

Life is not so simple for the compounding pharmacy, however, because creating medications takes multiple steps – and that could lead to errors in dosage, or the specific drug, or the percentages or dosage given. This is why BHRT practitioners should do due diligence in selecting a compounder to work with, and so should you. You need to find someone who takes quality and accuracy as seriously as you do. Only then can you expect the spectacular results we see with BHRT. The reason I advocate blood testing at regular intervals for patients on BHRT is a result of the nature of this process and the possibility of error. Blood testing is another way to ensure that the prescription written is the one that is dispensed. Safety also underlies my recommendation for practitioners to develop a close working relationship with a small number of competent, conscientious compounding pharmacies. In my experience, if your pharmacy takes quality as serious as you do, your results will be excellent.

Recently, U.S. pharmaceutical companies have been lobbying extensively to get the federal government to outlaw the compounding pharmacies. Their motto appears to be "If you can't compete with them, get rid of them." I can only hope common sense prevails, and this effort is unsuccessful. Good compounders take quality very seriously and go to great lengths to ensure it is job one.

WHERE TO FIND A COMPOUNDING PHARMACY

If you've already found your BHRT practitioner, then my advice is to use the compounding pharmacy he or she uses, because they've already developed a relationship, and the practitioner has experience with the quality of their work.

But if you're still looking for a BHRT practitioner in your area, a good way to start is to find a compounding pharmacist and ask who he or she works with. Try a Google search: Type the words "BHRT compounding pharmacy" and your city into the search box. That should give you a starting list. Then call two or three (or more) of the pharmacies on the list and ask for recommendations for BHRT practitioners. Check to see if the same names keep popping up.

You can also check out the International Academy of Compounding Pharmacists (IACP), an association that represents more than 2,000 compounding pharmacists. More than 87,000 patients and prescribers are also members. IACP provides a list of its member associations; you first must register at its website, http://www.iacprx.org/.

CHAPTER 17

YOUR PERSONALIZED PREVENTIVE-HEALTH PROGRAM

I hope by now I've made you a convert to the idea of BHRT and how it can help you to live a longer, healthier, happier life. Now we're going to explore how it all fits together for you – and how you can take the information you've learned and use it to improve and maintain your health, because that's really what it's all about!

We all recognize that as we age, our quality of life slowly deteriorates. This is probably one of the most often-voiced objections to the idea and science of significant life extension. The argument goes something like this: "What is the point of living longer if that means more years in a nursing home or as a house-confined senior?"

A lot of people aren't aware of exactly how much can be done – right now – to put more life in your years and more years in your life. And then there are rapidly developing technologies not even touched on here, but that will be able to yield significant life extension within the next 10 years.

Yes, I said within the next 10 years.

Back in Chapter 1, I mentioned the book *Fantastic Voyage* by Dr. Terry Grossman and Ray Kurzweil.

That book drove me to investigate this entire area of medicine. Fantastic Voyage outlines a near-term future very different from our reality today. Their concept of the exponential rate of technological change and development is seen around us every day. A cell phone 18 years ago was practically the size and weight of a brick. Compare that with today's cell phones.

The results of this accelerating rate of change are seen monthly in the health sciences. In fact, investment newsletters regularly highlight companies with products that would have seemed the stuff of Star Wars as little as 10 years ago.

As life extension occurs – and it will, whether we believe in it or not – it's in our best interest to use all the tools and resources at our disposal to develop and maintain the quality of life we want and deserve, especially because we have no control over the rate of accelerating change and the wide-ranging implications that will come with it.

I believe we will have many choices with respect to the technologies we use. And I also believe that those choices are going to explode in the coming decade. It has been said that when it comes to change, we overestimate how quickly a technology will come into common use and underestimate the effect of that technology on our lives.

Remember when the first personal computers were developed and how experts predicted a computer in every house within a few years? I can still remember one of my family members battling with an early floppy disk PC: You had to use one floppy disk to run the program, and then take it out and insert another disk to enter data. Progress seemed to take forever, and it was easy to wonder if computers would ever make a meaningful impact on day-to-day life. But just look at where we are now with the Internet and personal computing. Can you imagine most of us going through our day-to-day activities without the use of either?

This same wave of change is due to hit health care and life extension over the next 10 years. And since it's coming, we all might as well be in the best shape possible when it arrives.

Much of the improvement in quality of life starts with the basics. It is not possible to use only a BHRT program and ignore diet, exercise, stress reduction, sleep, and personal and work relationships and still achieve your optimal health.

I am not a guru, but I will do my best to give you some relevant observations about simple strategies and step-by-step measures you can take now. We'll also look at what supplements you can use and are readily available to improve your quality of life.

NUTRITION – YOU ARE WHAT YOU EAT

You now know that as we age, two of our hormones increase – namely cortisol and insulin. Their rise contributes to a state of accelerated aging. Dietary changes that reduce the levels of these two hormones contribute to healthy hormone balancing.

Consider this list of some of the problems caused by a rise in insulin levels:

- High blood pressure

- High cholesterol

- Weight gain

- Increased inflammation

Insulin levels are determined by our food choices, and are directly related to the balance of protein and sugar in our diet. Despite what some think, they are under our conscious control.

Without attention to diet, hormone balance is much more difficult – if not impossible. This association caused the American Journal of Cardiology to state in an editorial in 1972: "There is substantial evidence that changes in diet are responsible, in part, for the diseases that have emerged as dominant health problems in industrialized countries over the past century."

There are two basic hormones affected by dietary choices, insulin and glucagon.

Insulin rises as a result of sugar and simple-starch intake. Its job is to help maintain blood glucose levels within a narrow range. The brain is completely dependent on glucose for its energy needs. Too much or too little results in a critical problem for the brain, and the body has a complicated system to regulate glucose levels.

Simple starches and sugar in the diet are rapidly absorbed and cause blood sugar to spike. The pancreas responds by pouring out insulin to prevent the glucose levels from getting too high. Insulin works to transport blood glucose into fat cells for storage for a rainy day.

Unfortunately, insulin secretion overshoots the mark due to limitations in the system design, causing blood sugar to drop several hours after a meal of starch and simple sugars. The end result is a sugar craving, and if the food that satisfies that craving is available, the whole cycle starts all over again.

Glucagon is the body's natural antagonist to insulin, to bring balance to the equation. Protein in the diet causes secretion of glucagon, which causes stored sugar in the liver to be released. This raises blood sugar and glucagon directly reduces insulin secretion. If a meal is low in protein, it is usually high in starch and simple sugars.

So as you can see, dietary choices low in protein increase insulin levels and contribute directly to weight gain and increased inflammation. Each meal should have a portion of protein the size and thickness of your palm. This ensures adequate glucagon levels and low insulin levels, and contributes to consistent and steady weight loss. This is the basis of *The Zone Diet* by Dr. Barry Sears.

Your meal choices directly influence this powerful group of hormones: You truly are what you eat!

Our diets began to change in the 1960s with the debut of the low-fat diet. Eggs, bacon and other fatty foods were made out to be the enemy. Physicians, governments and food manufacturers wholeheartedly jumped on this bandwagon. Bacon and eggs was replaced with sugary cereals, and over time the obesity epidemic took off.

HIGH INSULIN'S VICIOUS CIRCLE

Elevated insulin serves as a hormone disruptor and antagonizes the actions of the other hormones. All the sex hormones are adversely affected, and, most important, so is thyroid hormone. The thyroid hormone establishes our metabolic rate and our ability to burn calories. High insulin disrupts thyroid conversion and results in a lower metabolic rate and even more weight gain.

Talk about a double whammy. As we gain weight, the harder it is for insulin to do its job, and we end up with a problem called insulin resistance. This means higher and higher levels of insulin are required to do the job – which leads to high blood pressure, high cholesterol, weight gain and inflammation.

But wait – it gets worse. Elevated insulin also stimulates cell growth, leading to an increased rate of cell division and telomere shortening. Telomeres are the ends of our chromosomes, much like the small end of a shoelace. Every time a cell divides, the telomeres on the chromosomes shorten. Most cells are equipped with telomeres long enough to allow only 17 divisions. After that, the telomeres will not allow further cell replication and that cell dies. At the present time, only daily supplementation with fish oil has been shown to reduce telomere shortening. There are, however, a number of drugs in development to do the same thing.

High insulin has many adverse effects in addition to easy weight gain. Recent studies have linked elevated insulin levels with an increased risk of cancer. We have long known about the link between obesity and cancer. Insulin may be the factor underlying obesity and cancer.

So how do we get off this potential train wreck? All activities directed at reducing insulin levels pay off in a multitude of benefits. The first step is to recognize the food-hormone connection. A reasonable portion of protein with each meal is essential. Carbohydrates should be in healthy forms, such as complex carbohydrates that do not aggravate the problems. Whole wheat and some of the old-style grains are more difficult for the body to convert directly into sugar. The slower the conversion, the less of an insulin spike is seen. Sugar in all of its obvious and disguised forms should be minimized.

I am not saying this is easy, but as a retired sugar-holic, I know it can be done. They say sugar is one of the most addictive substances we are exposed to and I heartily agree. I used to have two heaping teaspoons with my considerable number of coffees per day. Over time I was able to give up the addiction to sugar and found that time does decrease the cravings. In fact, the idea of a chocolate bar now seems disgusting, whereas years ago I considered it a dietary staple.

Colored and leafy vegetables grown above the ground are rich in antioxidants and have low caloric density.

Root vegetables in general are storage vessels for simple sugars and should be avoided because of their propensity to elevate blood glucose and insulin.

A plate should be one-third protein and the rest made up of a variety of healthy vegetables. Some fat is reasonable and certainly NOT the problem it has been made out to be.

A diet like this represents no hardship and should not be accompanied by hunger. You'll find all the good food choices on the outside aisles of the supermarket; avoid the inner aisles with their plethora of simple sugars and processed foods. Although I must say the industry is quick to adapt to simple axioms like this. A recent trip to a Florida supermarket revealed a lot of the unhealthier foods had been moved to the outside aisles. Organic foods are best, as they reduce the load of toxins and xenoestrogens that can also act as hormone disruptors.

There are many great books on food choices and the journey back to health. Two I have particularly enjoyed are Dr. Sears' *The Age Free Zone,* and *Hormone Harmony: How to Balance Insulin, Cortisol, Thyroid, Estrogen, Progesterone and Testosterone to Live Your Best Life* by Dr. Alicia Stanton. Both look closely at all aspects of the food-hormone connection and are highly recommended.

CORTISOL

The other twin horseman of accelerated aging is cortisol, the stress hormone that is vital to life and survival.

If protein intake is deficient, increased cortisol production ensures an adequate supply of blood glucose for the energy needs of the brain. If food is scarce, increased cortisol production causes the breakdown of muscle to provide a secondary source of glucose. Remember, no brain function, no survival!

Cortisol reduces the immediate effects of stress by interfering with eicosanoid signaling. Eicosanoids are the molecules of cell communication and a shutdown of their production is the ultimate hormone disruptor. Whenever I see adequate hormone levels in a patient on

BHRT and persisting adverse symptoms, stress is always at the base of the problem. We live in some of the most stressful times of history due to the rapid rate of change. Our bodies were not designed for this chronic type of stress and our health suffers as a result.

Chronically high levels of cortisol lead to numerous problems, including reduced immune function, loss of brain cells responsible for memory, reduced thyroid function, and lower metabolism. Poor eating habits – such as skipping breakfast – contribute to low blood glucose and elevated cortisol levels. Cortisol tears the body down, destroying muscle mass and contributing to accelerated aging. Decreased muscle mass destroys metabolism and contributes to weight gain and increased insulin levels.

One of the benefits of BHRT is its support of muscle mass. Normally as we age, we lose muscle mass secondary to gradually rising cortisol levels, a condition called sarcopenia. BHRT allows us to rebuild muscle with exercise and rejuvenate our metabolism. Remember, I did say BHRT is about much more than sex!

Besides improving our diets, other strategies help to reduce cortisol levels.

Meditation: This includes a variety of possibilities – activities such as yoga, transcendental meditation and Qi Gong. They are often overlooked, but can yield great benefits – especially if tied to visualization. We have a Qi Gong practitioner at our True Balance clinic and actively promote this form of meditation.

Moderate exercise: Start with the activities and hobbies you enjoy. It's interesting that the very activities we like the most can be nature's stress busters. Unfortunately, with the hectic pace of modern life, we often put the very pastimes that are good for us at the end of our priority lists. But this is counterproductive, when we look at the overall benefits provided through stress reduction. Remember, you don't have to do everything all at once. Try to make lifestyle changes over time that add items on your "love list" and weed out activities or duties that do not refresh you.

Good interpersonal relationships: Much has been said about this in other venues. But it's important to remember that, at the end of the day, it's only family and close friends who stick with us. There is no substitute for quality time with loved ones, spent in simple pleasures. I don't believe the recent trend toward cell phones and texting is a good one. To have good quality time, you need to be in the moment with those you are with. Many times I see people spending time together and yet really being elsewhere – because they're also on the phone or texting. This is a habit that must be fought continually. If nothing else, take some time every day and turn off the phone and just focus on being with the people who are most important to you. You can always retrieve your messages later. Do what you can to keep it real.

As mentioned earlier, high levels of cortisol also act to deplete progesterone and contribute to estrogen dominance. Progesterone is the building block for cortisol. If excess stress prevails, progesterone is diverted for extra cortisol production. Because cortisol is the hormone of survival, the need for it trumps progesterone requirements.

We can look at all the aspects of hormone balance as a kind of delicate spider's web – a change in one strand will be felt by all other areas of the system. By the same token, small changes in a positive direction are felt in many parts of the body. This leads to the concept of inner/outer balance.

YOUR "LOVE" LIST

If you're ready to begin working toward creating your own inner/outer balance, you might want to start a health/wellness journal. You could have a friend or partner quiz you by asking the following questions in rapid-fire succession (so you don't have time to think about them, but instead the answers come from the heart) and then make a list of your answers:

- What are the things you love to do?

- What are the activities that make your heart sing?

- What do you love?

- What do you love?

- What do you love?

Most people will have 15-20 "loves" before they run dry. The rapid-fire sequence is essential, as it circumvents the natural tendency to list the people or things in our life we "should" put on the list.

The next step is to look at your inner/outer (I/O) congruence. How much of what you love to do regularly shows up in your life? By making gradual changes in your life as decisions come up, you can move into a higher degree of I/O congruence and reduce your stress and cortisol levels.

EXERCISE

As I'm writing this section, I can almost hear myself groan. I am not a jock or a regular exerciser, but I do recognize this to be the next step in my longevity program. The food, lifestyle and hormone changes I have made in the last three years have me feeling better than I did 15 years ago. I believe there is even more improvement to come, in the form of a regular exercise program.

What's the big deal? Hormone balance with an overall shift to the anabolic side that results in the building up of our muscle mass is one of the fundamental benefits of BHRT. It increases the muscle-building sex hormones. Proper nutrition and stress-reduction techniques reduce insulin and cortisol levels. The net effect is a shift of body metabolism toward the rebuilding of muscle mass. Instead of a catabolic state where muscle is being steadily lost, we move to an anabolic state and the rebuilding of our muscle mass.

This re-establishes a healthy metabolic rate, further improves blood glucose and insulin levels, and directly opposes the progression of sarcopenia, which is so devastating in later life. Sarcopenia comes from the Greek and means "poverty of flesh" – it is the loss and degeneration of skeletal muscle mass that comes with aging.

Most people lose muscle mass as they age and become weak and prone to falls. If we are to live longer in total health, muscle mass must be preserved. An exercise program with a component of resistance or weight lifting exercise puts the reformation of our muscle mass into high gear.

But exercise is about much more than muscle mass. Regular exercise has dramatic and positive effects on brain function. This is critical, because what is the use of living longer if you forgot where you put your life? The research on the effects of exercise on learning and mood is exploding. The book *Spark: The Revolutionary New Science of Exercise and the Brain* by John Ratey is an excellent resource for those interested in a complete discussion of the area.

Regular exercise has been demonstrated to significantly increase a critical growth factor called brain derived neurotropic factor (BDNF). When I was in medical school, the popular thought was that the nervous system was nonplastic. That meant that whatever connections were made in childhood were fixed for the rest of life. It was believed that nerve cells could not divide or reproduce, and we were stuck with what we had. New research is turning the idea of a static nervous system upside down.

Most of it has to do with BDNF and its ability to maintain and build nervous system circuits. BDNF was discovered in 1990 and more than 10,000 articles have been written on this amazing compound.

A new fact, word or idea becomes part of our memory through a process called long-term potentiation (LTP). Learning involves a dynamic change in the activity between neurons. In a complicated process, new brain cell connections are developed and strengthened at the level of the individual synapse or cell-cell junction. BDNF is the main actor here and works through neuron gene activation to produce the changes that create new memories.

It was his work in this area that earned Dr. Eric Kandel of Columbia University the 2000 Nobel Prize for medicine. BDNF acts as the fertilizer for the development of new neuron connections – and exercise dramatically increases the levels of BDNF. More important, the increase in BDNF with exercise is most prominent in the hippo-campus, the area of our brain responsible for memory. BDNF is able to recruit neural stem cells at a dramatic rate. Studies with mice have shown a doubling of hippocampal stem cells in the mice that exercised as compared with their couch potato brothers and sisters.

VITAMIN D

It's really a misnomer to call this compound a vitamin. Vitamin D is truly a hormone in every sense of the word, and up to recently, it's been completely overlooked. Exposure to sunshine, just enough to slightly redden the skin, produces 20,000 units of Vitamin D in the body.

Fear of skin cancer and liberal use of sunscreens has lowered natural production of Vitamin D. Healthy sun exposure with the avoidance of sunburn doesn't increase the risk of skin cancer. In Canada, we have an epidemic of Vitamin D deficiency that has a number of important negative effects on our health.

Supplementation with 2,000-6,000 units of Vitamin D daily, followed up by a blood measurement to document adequate levels, is critical to your health. Achieving a level of 120 mmol/l in the blood produces a 50% reduction in breast, colon, pancreatic and prostate cancer.

The most prestigious medical journal in North America, *The New England Journal of Medicine*, reported these facts in 2007[1], but change in physician attitudes is slow.

What other simple supplement can produce such a dramatic reduction in cancer rates? It is impossible to overdose on 2,000 units even with sun exposure, and some people will need up to and above 5,000 units per day to get adequate levels. There is also strong evidence that optimal levels of Vitamin D improve mental function and mood, protect against heart disease, and prevent Alzheimer's disease. Vitamin D is inexpensive, readily available, and should be part of everyone's preventative health program.

OMEGA 3'S

Omega oils are the long-chain fatty acids in our diet that are incorporated into the membranes of every cell of our body. Think of your cell membranes in terms of a large warehouse needed for a business to function. The racks of the warehouse are filled with omega 3 and 6 compounds. The ratio of the two to each other determines the compounds most likely to be used. Omega 3s direct cell metabolism toward a state of low inflammation and omega 6s are the opposite. Now multiply this process over the 1 trillion cells in your body and you can get a glimpse of how important this omega 3/6 ratio can be.

Omega 3s are found in fish and fish oil; they are very beneficial and act to reduce inflammation. Omega 6s are found in processed food and directly increase levels of inflammation in the body. Omega 6s are metabolized to arachidonic acid (AA), a very powerful mediator of inflammatory prostaglandins in the body. AA production is increased with high levels of insulin, and high insulin levels are seen with obesity. This is one of the paths obesity uses to increase inflammation in the body. Omega 3s block the production of AA, and turn the cell metabolism toward the production of inflammation-reducing prostaglandins.

Prostaglandins are the body's messengers, spreading the word about what's happening. Inflammation is bad and can be measured with the C-reactive protein (CRP) level. CRP is always measured at the beginning of a BHRT program to help us decide where we need to start. This is important because of the relationship between increased levels of inflammation and heart disease. CRP has become an established risk factor for heart disease as we have learned about the connection between increased inflammation and heart disease.

Heart disease is much more than just a lipid problem[2]. Hundreds of years ago, we had a healthy balance of roughly 1:6 between omega 3s and 6s. That changed with the introduction of processed food, and the ratio is now about 1:25. This increased ratio is one of the many problems caused by our compromised food supply.

To raise levels of omega 3s, everyone should take a pharmaceutical fish oil supplement at a dose of 2 grams per day. Fish oil has two important components: EPA and DHA. DHA is critical for proper brain development and function. Studies have shown omega 3 supplementation to be effective in the treatment of attention deficit disorder and depression. EPA appears to be critical for elasticity and proper function of the lining of our blood vessels. When this lining, the endothelium, is healthy, it keeps inflammation levels low and promotes health. In general, 2 grams of good quality fish oil will yield 1200 mg of combined EPA and DHA.

You can check the side of the bottle to calculate the combined level of these two compounds. Pharmaceutical grade means the fish oil is of guaranteed potency and is free of mercury and dioxin. Once you are on the recommended dose of fish oil, it is possible to test your blood to ensure the dose is optimal for you. Private labs can do an AA/

EPA ratio, with the target being a ratio of 1.5-4.5. This ratio reduces the risk of death by 25% over five years.

And on top of that, an optimal AA/EPA ratio improves brain and heart health[3], and has been shown to reduce formation of tumor necrosis factor-alpha (TNF), a powerful mediator of inflammation in the body.

Omega 3 supplementation has been shown to reduce breast cancer risk[4] and have beneficial effects on the symptoms of rheumatoid arthritis[5]. There is also new evidence that omega 3 supplementation slows telomere shortening, a critical indicator of remaining cell multiplication potential. Increased telomere length is directly related to expected longevity and can now be measured.

MULTIVITAMINS

Everyone has a different idea of what constitutes a good multivitamin. As changes in our food supply have degraded the quality and amounts of nutrients in what we eat, vitamin supplementation has become more important. Traditionally, vitamins were suggested in doses to meet recommended daily allowances (RDA), levels below which disease can be predicted to occur in a person. RDAs are an antiquated concept that must be discarded.

Many vitamins are part of the body's defense mechanism against oxidative damage or "rusting." Oxidative damage is secondary to inefficiencies of energy production and damages cell walls, enzymes and our DNA.

Over the millennia, a complicated defense mechanism developed with many redundancies to protect against oxidative damage. Agents such as glutathione, alpha-lipoic acid, and Vitamins A, B, C, D and E all work in concert to recycle one another and to eliminate free radicals.

Modern medicine still does not recognize the synergy between these compounds and continues to study individual vitamins rather than the entire chain. Looking at these compounds through the RDA glass gives an incomplete idea of the importance they play in prevention of oxidative damage.

Plants evolved over the millennia exposed to high levels of oxidative damage from sunlight. Plants can't move to get away from the sun and need it for their growth. They developed complicated mechanisms involving bioflavanoids and polyphenol compounds to combat oxidative damage. In my opinion, a good multivitamin delivers optimal levels of the known vitamins as well as protective levels of the plant-based products.

These vitamins are not found over the counter in your local drugstore. Like most things in life, you get what you pay for. Good multivitamins are a little more expensive and require the user to take four to nine per day.

I am not a fan of measuring vitamin levels in the body; I prefer to measure indicators of oxidative damage. Private labs have developed a sophisticated panel of tests to measure an individual's levels of oxidative damage. The result is a quantitation of the net effects of diet, exercise, lifestyle and supplement in an individual and takes into account his or her genetic makeup. What better way to look at the effectiveness of a particular vitamin program? Any practitioner with training in functional and regenerative medicine will be able to access this testing.

You've probably picked up a common theme: Make changes and MEASURE the effects in yourself to ensure the desired result has been achieved. If not, change the program and remeasure that indicator till you get it right!

MAGNESIUM AND TOXICITY

Proper bowel function is essential; it allows us to get rid of toxins and chemicals that would otherwise clog up our systems: These toxins are found in our food, water and environment. Toxicity is starting to gain more visibility and is well covered in Dr. S. Rogers' book *Detoxify or Die*.

The liver has a diverse array of enzymes that can render these noxious agents harmless. Once a toxin is inactivated by the liver, the body secretes it into the bowel. Regular bowel movements facilitate elimination of the toxins.

Proper bowel function depends on adequate levels of fiber in the diet. Processed foods are low in fiber, and constipation is a common condition today. The sign of a well-functioning bowel is a soft bowel movement once or twice per day. If this does not happen, detoxification is impaired and toxins are likely to be reabsorbed into the body. These toxins act as cellular poisons and should be minimized.

In addition to increasing fiber, magnesium supplementation can often work miracles to restore healthy bowel function. Magnesium is a critical cofactor in approximately 500 enzyme reactions and is a very important balance to the effects of calcium at the cellular level.

Doses of 250-750 mg/day of magnesium will often produce regular bowel habits even in those who have never had proper function. Overdose results in diarrhea and is easily reversed by reducing the dose. Research has shown that approximately half of North Americans are magnesium-deficient. In addition to constipation, other symptoms of magnesium deficiency include chocolate cravings, depression, PMS, headaches, low energy, restless leg syndrome, insomnia, and poor nail growth.

Magnesium is also critical to proper bone metabolism and heart and blood vessel function. *Detoxify or Die* covers the whole area of detoxification very thoroughly, and it's a book I recommend.

It's also critical to avoid or minimize toxin exposure. Ion foot baths and regular infrared sauna treatments can also greatly assist the detoxification process.

COENZYME Q10

CoQ10 is found in every cell and is essential for the production of energy. It works at the level of the mitochondria, the little fuel cells found in every cell. CoQ10 levels start to decline at age 35 and contribute to heart disease and low energy.

Heart cells have the highest concentration of mitochondria in the body, as they sustain the energy requirements of the heart to keep us alive. Numerous studies have shown that CoQ10 improves symptoms of angina, congestive heart failure, and other diseases of the heart muscle.

CoQ10 also appears to play a role in cell growth and protects against damage that can lead to cancer.

CoQ10 comes in two forms, ubiquinone and ubiquinol. Ubiquinol is the reduced form of CoQ10 and is much more active than its counterpart. Supplementation with 120 mg/day is an essential part of a preventative health program.

RESVERATROL

The story of this compound is one of the most fascinating. Only recently discovered, resveratrol is one of a group of compounds called sirtuins, or silent information regulating transcription compounds. At the present time, the only intervention that has been proven to extend life is caloric restriction.

A 15% reduction in calorie intake below what is needed for caloric neutrality gives a 25% increase in lifespan. This has been proven in mice and observational studies in humans are in agreement. Studies of survivors of some of the terrible famines in the 20th century confirm increased life expectancy in these individuals. Caloric restriction reduces oxidative damage, blood glucose and insulin levels. These effects conspire to significantly extend life expectancy. But, it remains an unpopular approach in these times of plentiful food.

If the body is forced to adapt to conditions where not enough calories are present it does some fancy recalibration. Since it takes calories to reproduce and what is the point of producing a child in a

famine, caloric restriction shuts down the gene expression for reproduction. Genes are activated to try to increase longevity in hopes of
surviving to a time of caloric plenty. Caloric restriction modifies the
expression of approximately 2,000 genes with the net effect of significant life extension.

Plant-based resveratrol does the same thing, without the maintain
caloric restriction.

A plant has two basic choices in life, reproduction or growth.
Reproduction requires a significant expenditure of energy and needs
to be carefully controlled. Over time, plants developed a mechanism
to signal external environmental events via sirtuins. In drought or
other hostile conditions, sirtuins are produced to divert plant energy
into growth and away from reproduction. Why bother flowering in a
drought only to have the seeds die?

Over the millennia, because we animals share the same biosphere,
humans developed sensitivity for these sirtuins. As in the plants,
increased sirtuin levels direct energy utilization toward growth and
preservation of the individual: It is better to live to reproduce in a more
favorable environment.

It is believed that sirtuins are at least partially responsible for the
"French paradox," which was the observation of lifestyle and longevity
in the French in days gone by. A rich diet accompanied by daily red
wine intake did not result in the expected incidence of heart disease
and death. Don't try this with today's red wine; sufficient intake would
relegate you to the life of an alcoholic. The grapevines of yesteryear
often had fungal infections that stressed the plants and increased sirtuin
production.

Resveratrol is the first of many of these sirtuins to become available. Expect to hear much more about these compounds in the future. The recommended dose of optimized trans-resveratrol is 250 mg/day.

BIOIDENTICAL HORMONES

I hope that you understand now how BHRT can fit into your own longevity program. I've done my best to lay out the evidence for you.

BHRT is about much more than sex or compounding "witchcraft." We now have the ability to re-engineer the hormone system of the body using the native, natural hormones. Our future years are not predestined to be characterized by declining function and reduced enjoyment.

BHRT is safe and can be individualized for you on the basis of symptoms, in order to improve your quality of life. What's more, it can be measured to ensure that safe physiologic levels are achieved.

Simple steps can be used to re-establish the healthy hormone balance we had in our 20s.

As exciting as these times are, we are still stumbling in the dark with respect to longevity extension. New technologies will, in our lifetimes, allow the monitoring and maintenance of these hormones and vitamins in real time. It may be a Star Trek view, but I truly believe the future is closer than you think. I wish you good health and much love and happiness in the future.

1 NEJM; 2007; 357; 266-81 M. Hoflick / 2 Am J Clin Nutr 2008; 87s; 1997s-2002s W Harris / 3 Preventative Medicine 2004; 39; 212-20 W Harris et al. / 4 Am J Clin Nutr 2008; 87s; 1997s-2002s W Harris / 5 Seminars in Arthritis and Rheumatism 1997; 27; 2; 85-97 M James et al.

For more inforamtion on Medical Grade Aesthetics and
Bioidentical Hormone Replacement Therapy (BHRT),
please visit my website at:
mytruebalance.ca